School Nursing

3rd Edition

Scope and Standards of Practice

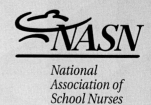

National
Association of
School Nurses

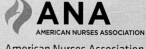

AMERICAN NURSES ASSOCIATION

American Nurses Association
Silver Spring, Maryland 2017

American Nurses Association
8515 Georgia Avenue, Suite 400
Silver Spring, MD 20910-3492
1-800-274-4ANA
http://www.Nursingworld.org

The American Nurses Association (ANA) is the only full-service professional organization representing the interests of the nation's 3.6 million registered nurses through its constituent member nurses associations and its organizational affiliates. ANA advances the nursing profession by fostering high standards of nursing practice, promoting the rights of nurses in the workplace, projecting a positive and realistic view of nursing, and lobbying the Congress and regulatory agencies on healthcare issues affecting nurses and the public.

The American Nurses Association (ANA) and National Association of School Nurses (NASN) are national professional associations. This ANA–NASN publication, *School Nursing: Scope and Standards of Practice, 3rd Edition*, reflects the thinking of the nursing profession on various issues and should be reviewed in conjunction with state board of nursing policies and practices. State law, rules, and regulations govern the practice of nursing, while *School Nursing: Scope and Standards of Practice, 3rd Edition*, guides nurses in the application of their professional knowledge, skills, and responsibilities.

ISBN-13: 978-1-55810-719-9   SAN: 851-3481   06/2017
eISBNs: 978-1-55810-692-5 (ePDF) ... 978-1-55810-693-2 (EPUB) ...
        978-1-55810-694-9 (Kindle)
First printing: June 2017

Contents

Contributors

NASN Work Group Members

Cheryl-Ann Resha, EdD, MSN, RN, FNASN (Chair)—Connecticut

Editor and Standards Task Force Leader, *School Nursing: Scope and Standards of Practice*, 2017; member of Standards Task Force, 2011; professor of nursing, Southern Connecticut State University; current National Association of School Nurses Board member (Connecticut Representative); past president and past treasurer, National Association of State School Nurse Consultants; past school nurse supervisor, West Hartford, Connecticut.

Elizabeth Chau, SRN (UK), RN—Washington, DC

School nurse (retired), Washington, DC; immediate past executive Board member, National Association of School Nurses (NASN); immediate past NASN Board Member (DC Representative); immediate past chair Private and Parochial School Nurse (PPSN), Special Interest Group (SIG) of NASN.

Julia Muennich Cowell, PhD, APHN-BS, FAAN—California

Executive editor, *The Journal of School Nursing*; member, Standards Task Force, 2005, 2011; professor emerita, College of Nursing, Rush University, Chicago, Illinois.

Saria Lofton, PhD, RN—Chicago

Assistant professor, College of Nursing, University of Illinois at Chicago, Chicago, Illinois.

Dianne Mennitt, DNP, MS, BSN, RN, PHCNS-BC, AE-C, NCSN—Florida

State school nurse consultant, University of South Florida Student Support Services Project, Florida Department of Education, Tallahassee, Florida; member of the National Association of State School Nurse Consultants (NASSNC).

Mary E. Newell, PhD, RN, NCSN—Washington

Coordinator for Nursing and Health Services, Kent School District, Kent, Washington.

Susan Nokleby, MS, RN, LSN, NCSN—Minnesota

President, School Nurse Organization of Minnesota; past president, National Board for Certification of School Nurses; Johnson and Johnson School Health Leadership Fellow; school nurse, Intermediate School District 287, Minnetonka, Minnesota.

Cescilee Rall, BSN, RN, NCSN—Utah

Past president, Utah School Nurses Association; chair, Utah State Board of Nursing; secondary lead school nurse, Granite School District, Salt Lake City, Utah.

Rhoda Shepherd, MA, BSN, RN, FNASN—Iowa

Past secretary-treasurer, National Association of School Nurses; past Board and Executive Board member, Nominating Committee Member, National Association of School Nurses; past president, Iowa School Nurse Organization; former school nurse, manager health services, and director student services (retired), Cedar Rapids Community School District, Cedar Rapids, Iowa.

Elizabeth L. Thomas, MEd, BS, RN, NCSN, FNASN—Delaware

Past editor and Standards Task Force Leader, *School Nursing: Scope and Standards of Practice*, 2005 and 2011; past Board and Executive Board member, National Association of School Nurses; chair, ANA *Nursing: Scope and Standards of Practice*, 2015; past president, Delaware School Nurse Association; school nurse and school nurse coordinator (retired), Wilmington, Delaware; consultant, School Health Consulting.

ANA Staff

Carol J. Bickford, PhD, RN-BC, CPHIMS, FHIMSS, FAAN – Content editor

Joi Morris, BS, CAP-OM – Project coordinator

Lisa M. Myers, Esq. – Legal counsel

Liz Stokes, JD, RN – Ethics consultant

Eric Wurzbacher, BA – Project editor

ANA Committee on Nursing Practice Standards

Renee Gecsedi, MS, RN, Co-Chair

Danette Culver, MSN, APRN, ACNS-BC, CCRN, Co-Chair

Patricia Bowe, DNP, MS, RN

Deedra Harrington, DNP, APRN, ACNP-BC

Richard Henker, PhD, RN, CRNA, FAAN, Co-Chair

Maria Jurlano, MS, RN, NEA-BC, CCRN

Tonette McAndrew, MPA, BSN, RN

Verna Sitzer, PhD, RN, CNS

Carla Lee, PhD, APRN-BC, CNAA, FAAN, FIBA, Alternate

Tom Blodgett, PhD, MSN, RN-BC, Alternate

About the National Association of School Nurses

The National Association of School Nurses (NASN) is a nonprofit specialty nursing organization, organized in 1968 and incorporated in 1977, representing school nurses exclusively. NASN has over 15,000 members and 51 affiliates, including in the District of Columbia and overseas. The mission of the NASN is "to improve the health and educational success of children and youth by developing and providing leadership to advance the school nursing practice."

About the American Nurses Association

The American Nurses Association (ANA) is the only full-service professional organization representing the interests of the nation's 3.6 million registered nurses through its constituent member nurses associations and its organizational affiliates. ANA advances the nursing profession by fostering high standards of nursing practice, promoting the rights of nurses in the workplace, projecting a positive and realistic view of nursing, and lobbying the Congress and regulatory agencies on healthcare issues affecting nurses and the public.

Preface

The scope and standards of school nursing practice provide a mechanism of accountability of the specialty to the public. The scope describes the who, what, where, when, how, and why of the specialty practice. Standards are professional expectations that guide the practice of school nursing. The standards have practical and formal value in advocacy, decision-making, setting and describing professional values and roles, and framing issues that "connote a norm, establish an expectation, and facilitate measurement" (Proctor, in Selekman, 2013, p. 49). Meeting the standards and associated competencies provides evidence of a standard of care. Used as a framework, the scope and standards of school nursing practice describe the core of the specialty.

Relationship of School Nursing's Foundational Documents

A critical resource for professional nursing practice is *Nursing: Scope and Standards of Practice, 3rd Edition* (ANA, 2015b). This foundational document describes the comprehensive practice of nursing, outlines the expectations of the professional role of the registered nurse, and presents the Standards of Professional Nursing Practice for all registered nurses with accompanying competencies. It is the document on which this description of the specialty practice of school nursing, *School Nursing: Scope and Standards of Practice, 3rd Edition*, is based. The scope and standards of school nursing describe a competent level of school nursing practice and professional performance.

Registered nurses, practicing as school nurses, whether in the United States or abroad for the U.S. Department of Defense Education Activity, also have other key professional resources that inform their thinking and decision-making and guide their practice. *Code of Ethics for Nurses with Interpretive Statements* (ANA, 2015a) and its companion, *Guide to the Code of Ethics for Nurses: Development, Interpretation and Application, 2nd Edition* (Fowler, 2015) assist in ethical decision-making. These documents set the ethical framework for registered nurses across all roles, levels, and settings. School nurses are further advised by the 2016 edition of *Code of Ethics with Interpretive Statements for the School Nurse* published by the National Association of School Nurses.

Audience

School nurses, school nurse administrators, and registered nurses are the primary audience of this professional resource. Healthcare providers, healthcare systems, agencies and organizations, other nursing specialties (such as public health nurses), school district administrators, school board members, and interprofessional colleagues will also find this a valuable reference in understanding the role of school nurses, the supervision of nursing personnel and unlicensed assistive personnel in schools, and the development, maintenance, and evaluation of the school health program. In addition, students, families, groups, communities, and other populations using healthcare services in the school and in the community can use this document to better understand what comprises the practice of school nursing provided by registered nurses, advanced practice registered nurses, and graduate-level-prepared school nurses. Finally, legislators, regulators, legal counsel, and the judiciary system may wish to reference this document describing the scope of school nursing practice and the accompanying specialty standards of practice and professional performance.

Scope of School Nursing Practice

Definitions and Distinguishing Characteristics of School Nursing Practice

Definitions

Nursing is the protection, promotion, and optimization of health and abilities, prevention of illness and injury, facilitation of healing, alleviation of suffering through the diagnosis and treatment of human response, and advocacy in the care of individuals, families, groups, communities, and populations (ANA, 2015b, p. 1).

School nursing, a specialized practice of nursing, protects and promotes student health, facilitates optimal development, and advances academic success. School nurses, grounded in ethical and evidence-based practice, are the leaders who bridge health care and education, provide care coordination, advocate for quality student-centered care, and collaborate to design systems that allow individuals and communities to develop their full potential (National Association of School Nurses [NASN], 2017).

The definitions of nursing and school nursing provide the base for the unique specialty scope and standards of school nursing practice.

Distinguishing Characteristics

The *Framework for 21st Century School Nursing Practice* (NASN, 2016c) characterizes the student as the central focus of care and highlights the principles guiding school nursing practice that are evident in the Standards of School Nursing Practice. The principles include care coordination, leadership, quality improvement (QI), and community/public health. The principles are not hierarchical but overlap and are conceived to be synergistic. The components of each of the principles reflect nursing activities that enhance the entire school community's health and well-being. For example, care coordination requires leadership skills that are systems level in order to advocate for optimal population health and wellness. Care coordination is continuously analyzed in programs to ensure QI. In addition, effective care coordination assures students access to care, thus addressing the public's health (NASN, 2016c).

The *Framework for 21st Century School Nursing Practice* is congruent with *Nursing's Social Policy Statement* (American Nurses Association [ANA], 2010), long considered a foundational document for nursing practice that identified the following ". . . essential features of contemporary nursing practice":

- Provision of a caring relationship that facilitates health and healing
- Attention to the range of human experiences and responses to health and illness in the physical and social environments
- Integration of assessment data with knowledge gained from an appreciation of the patient or group
- Application of scientific knowledge to the processes of diagnosis and treatment through the use of judgment and critical thinking
- Advancement of professional nursing knowledge through scholarly inquiry
- Influence on social and public policy to promote social justice
- Assurance of safe, quality and evidence-based practice (p. 9).

School Nursing's Scope and Standards of Practice
Description of the Scope of School Nursing Practice

The scope of practice statement describes the "who," "what," "where," "when," "how," and "why" of school nursing practice. Each of these questions must be sufficiently answered to provide a complete picture of the dynamic and complex practice of school nursing and its evolving and expanding boundaries.

According to the ANA (2015b):

> The definition of nursing provides a succinct characterization of the "what" of nursing. Registered nurses and advanced practice registered nurses comprise the "who" and have been educated, titled, and maintain active licensure to practice nursing. Nursing occurs "when" ever there is a need for nursing knowledge, wisdom, caring, leadership, practice, or education, anytime, anywhere. Nursing occurs in any environment "where" there is a healthcare consumer in need of care, information, or advocacy. The "how" of nursing practice is defined as the ways, means, methods, and manners that nurses use to practice professionally. The "why" is characterized as nursing's response to the changing needs of society to achieve

positive healthcare consumer outcomes in keeping with nursing's social contract with an obligation to society (p. 2).

The following definitions clarify the role of a school nurse:

- *Who.* Recommended to be a registered, professional nurse with at least a baccalaureate degree in nursing (bachelor of science in nursing [BSN]) from an accredited college or university, as well as state certification in those states requiring or recommending state school nurse licensure/certification. School nurses provide individual and population-based care as generalists or specialists. The role of school nurse is unique and varied and may include clinician, advocate, counselor, educator, liaison, care coordinator, collaborator, interprofessional team member, student services case manager, researcher, administrator, leader, and others. For more details on this role, go to the section starting on pg. 27.

- *What.* A specialty practice of professional nursing that, in collaboration with families, school personnel, and other healthcare providers, is responsible for the health and well-being of school students and the school community, generally in the pre-kindergarten to Grade 12 setting. For more details on this role, go to the section starting on pg. 10.

- *Where.* Usually within a school setting, which may extend beyond the physical building to include the school community, off-campus school trips, and athletic events. School nurses may be employed in an advisory or managerial capacity by boards of education, public health agencies, healthcare institutions, and within the federally funded school system of the Department of Defense Education Activity (DoDEA) in the United States and around the world. For more details on this role, go to the section starting on pg. 20.

- *When.* Generally during regularly scheduled school hours, and in extended coverage locations, such as boarding/residential schools and detention centers. The school nurse may also be asked to be "on call" or provide nursing services during times when the students are participating in off-campus field trips or work experiences. For more details on this role, go to the section starting on pg. 25.

- *Why.* To support the health, well-being, and the ultimate educational success and lifelong achievement of students in keeping with the social contract of nursing. For more details on this role, go to the section starting on pg. 33.

- *How.* Guided by a caring and strong ethical code, using a culturally congruent and holistic approach to the nursing process, and in keeping with nursing's commitment to society. School nurses integrate the five core healthcare professional practice competencies (student-centered practice, evidence-based practice, interprofessional collaboration, use of informatics, continuous quality improvement) to provide effective, comprehensive communication and advance the profession of nursing by facilitating the protection of vulnerable subjects (students) when conducting and sharing research (Institute of Medicine [IOM], 2003). For more details on this role, go to the section starting on pg. 13.

The specialty of school nursing encompasses a broad range of nursing responsibilities and settings. The depth and breadth in which individual school nurses engage in the total scope of school nursing practice depend on their education, licensure, experience, role, work environment and workload, and the population served.

About the Standards of School Nursing Practice
Origin of School Nursing Standards

Professional nursing and nursing specialty organizations have a responsibility to their members and to the public they serve to develop standards of practice. As the professional organization for all registered nurses (RNs), the ANA has assumed the responsibility for developing standards that apply to the practice of all RNs and serve as a template for the development of school nursing standards as specialty standards. ANA (2015b) suggests that "Competencies in individual specialty areas of practice may be defined by separate specialty scope and standards documents authored by specialty nursing associations" (p. 38). Hence, as a specialty organization representing school nurses, the National Association of School Nurses (NASN) has been developing and promoting the scope and standards of school nursing practice since 1983.

History of School Nursing Standards

Standards of professional school nursing practice pertain to the specialty practice of school nursing. Throughout the early and mid-20th century, many school nurses and professional nursing groups attempted to define school nursing and articulate roles and functions, both essential to the development of standards (Appendix A). Others outside of nursing also weighed in. Reflective of the considerable paternalism of the day, a joint committee of the National Education Association (NEA) and the American Medical Association (1941) authored a paper titled *The Nurse in the School* that defined and established a role for nursing in schools.

By 1960, no fewer than five groups were speaking for school nursing: the School Nurses Branch, Public Health Nursing Section of the ANA; the

Committee on School Nursing Policies and Practices of the American School Health Association; Public Health Nurses Section of the America Public Health Association; National Council for School Nurses of the American Association for Health, Physical Education and Recreation; and the Department of School Nurses of the NEA, representing the majority of school nurses. These groups authored significant papers on the role and function of school nursing (Appendix A). By 1970, the Department of School Nurses of the NEA, later to become NASN, had grown in influence among school nurses and published a role and function paper of its own (NEA Department of School Nurses, 1970).

In 1983, after eight decades of identifying and refining the role of the school nurse, the first national standards of practice were developed when several organizations, all interested in school nursing, came together under the leadership and direction of NASN to produce a set of standards modeled on a template laid down by the ANA (1983). The 2017 document, *School Nursing: Scope and Standards of Practice, Third Edition*, is the latest set of published school nursing standards using an ANA-stipulated format and describing a competent level of nursing practice and professional performance common to and expected of all school nurses.

Development and Function of School Nursing Standards

The Standards of School Nursing Practice accompany the Scope of School Nursing Practice. The Standards of School Nursing Practice are authoritative statements of the duties that school nurses, regardless of role, are expected to perform competently (adapted from ANA, 2015b, p. 3). The standards published herein may serve as evidence of the standard of care, with the understanding that with the wide range of roles and functions of a school nurse, application of the standards is dependent upon individual job description and practice setting (McDaniel, Overman, Guttu, & Engelke, 2013).

The dynamics of the school nursing specialty require standards to be updated and revised. As expectations for the academic success and lifelong achievement of students evolve, and changes in societal trends occur, school nursing, the education community, and the public will develop and accept new patterns of professional practice. In response, nursing standards must have "formal, periodic review and revision" (ANA, 2015b, p. 3). NASN assumes this responsibility for the specialty of school nursing and completed the review and revision of *School Nursing: Scope and Standards of Practice, 2nd Edition* (2011).

This third edition document includes 20 standards statements that serve school nurses and school communities as a framework for outlining an expansive scope of practice. The language is intentionally broad and serves to paint an overall picture of practice. The standards statements, upon further development and explication, become more effective as a comprehensive and refined listing of expectations essential to practice. Furthermore, "the roles and activities in which the school nurse engages, particularly as the nurse uses the nursing process, may be state and/or district specific, and the uniqueness of a given position cannot be fully understood, comprehended, or appreciated through the use of standards statements by themselves. Standards statements, therefore, optimally serve nursing practice or the recipients of nursing care when further tailored to the specifics of the focus or setting" (Proctor, in Selekman, 2013, p. 50).

Each standard's statement is accompanied by several basic competencies. The competency statements, in turn, may be further specified as befits the practice setting. The competencies described for the generalist school nurse are applicable to all school nurses. Additional competencies may be identified for the graduate-level-prepared school nurse and for the advanced practice registered nurse (APRN). Competencies are specific, measurable elements that interpret, explain, and facilitate practical use of a standard. The competencies may be evidence of compliance with the individual standard but are not exhaustive and depend on the circumstances. McDaniel et al. (2013) demonstrate how school nursing competencies associated with the Standards guide the evaluation of school nurse performance by providing evidence of completed activities. Competencies may be used by school nursing professionals to appraise professional performance and to provide a clearer understanding of the role of the school nurse to school administrators, faculty, staff, and the entire school community (Haffke, Damm, & Cross, 2014). School nurses can identify opportunities for development and improvement of their practice by self-evaluation based on competency statements.

Overview of the Standards of School Nursing Practice

The Standards of School Nursing Practice consist of Standards of Practice and Standards of Professional Performance. The Standards of Practice are the six steps of the nursing process. The use of the nursing process as standards represents the directive nature of the standards as the school nurse completes each component of the nursing process. Similarly, the standards of professional performance relate to how the school nurse adheres to all the standards of practice and addresses other nursing practice issues, concerns, and activities. Together, the Standards of Practice and the Standards of Professional Performance provide authoritative statements that all school nurses perform competently. These standards provide evidence of a standard of care and do depend on context, especially in unusual situations (adapted from ANA, 2015b, p. 3).

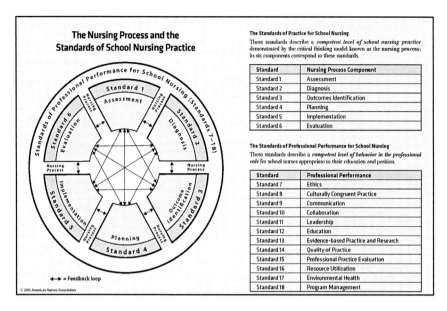

Figure 1. The nursing process and the Standards of Practice for School Nursing (adapted from ANA, 2015b, pp. 14–15).

Standards of Practice for School Nursing

The Standards of Practice for School Nursing describe a competent level of nursing care as demonstrated by the critical thinking model known as the nursing process. These standards encompass all significant actions taken by school nurses and form the foundation of the school nurse's decision-making (ANA, 2015b, p. 4). The Standards of Practice model in Figure 1 demonstrates that the six elements are not linear, but interactive and multidirectional as the school nurse uses and reuses the nursing process in practice.

The Standards of Practice for School Nursing are as follows:

Standard 1. Assessment

The school nurse collects pertinent data and information relative to the student's health or the situation.

Standard 2. Diagnosis

The school nurse analyzes the assessment data to determine actual or potential diagnoses, problems, and issues.

Standard 3. Outcomes Identification

The school nurse identifies expected outcomes for a plan individualized to the student or the situation.

Standard 4. Planning

The school nurse develops a plan that prescribes strategies to attain expected, measurable outcomes.

Standard 5. Implementation

The school nurse implements the identified plan.

Standard 5a. Coordination of Care

The school nurse coordinates care delivery.

Standard 5b. Health Teaching and Health Promotion

The school nurse employs strategies to promote health and a safe environment.

Standard 6. Evaluation

The school nurse evaluates progress toward attainment of goals and outcomes.

Standards of Professional Performance for School Nursing

The Standards of Professional Performance for School Nursing describe a competent level of behavior in the professional role. All school nurses are expected to actively engage in professional role activities appropriate to their education, experience, and position. School nurses are accountable for their professional actions to themselves, their students, families, and school communities; the profession; and, ultimately, to society (adapted from ANA, 2015b, p. 5).

The Standards of Professional Performance for School Nursing are as follows:

Standard 7. Ethics

The school nurse practices ethically.

Standard 8. Culturally Congruent Practice

The school nurse practices in a manner that is congruent with cultural diversity and inclusion principles.

Standard 9. Communication

The school nurse communicates effectively in all areas of practice.

Standard 10. Collaboration

The school nurse collaborates with key stakeholders in the conduct of nursing practice.

Standard 11. Leadership

The school nurse leads within the professional practice setting and the profession.

Standard 12. Education

The school nurse seeks knowledge and competence that reflects current nursing practice and promotes futuristic thinking.

Standard 13. Evidence-Based Practice and Research

The school nurse integrates evidence and research findings into practice.

Standard 14. Quality of Practice

The school nurse contributes to quality nursing practice.

Standard 15. Professional Practice Evaluation

The school nurse evaluates one's own and others' nursing practice.

Standard 16. Resource Utilization

The school nurse utilizes appropriate resources to plan, provide, and sustain evidence-based nursing services that are safe, effective, and fiscally responsible.

Standard 17. Environmental Health

The school nurse practices in an environmentally safe and healthy manner.

Standard 18. Program Management

The school nurse directs the health services program within the school and community that includes evidence-based practice and accountability measures for quality, student health and learning outcomes.

The What of School Nursing

What is school nursing?

School nursing, a specialized practice of nursing, protects and promotes student health, facilitates optimal development, and advances academic success. School nurses, grounded in ethical and evidence-based practice, are the leaders who bridge health care and education, provide care coordination, advocate for quality student-centered care, and collaborate to design systems that allow individuals and communities to develop their full potential (NASN, 2017).

School nursing is guided by the principles of care coordination, leadership, quality improvement, and community/public health and supported by the overarching tenets of school nursing practice.

The role of the school nurse is unique because it encompasses both community health nursing and public health nursing responsibilities in the educational setting. Community health nursing focuses on the individual in the community and subsequently influences the community, while public health nursing focuses on the population and consequently influences the individual. The combined responsibilities require competencies that are focused equally on the care of the individual and the general population.

More than 100 years ago, public health nurse founder Lillian Wald envisioned a role for the nurse within the community to serve all, regardless of economic or social status or national origin. Early disease prevention in public health focused on exclusion of students with infection. The modern framework encourages the inclusion of children with chronic illness in the school setting (primarily pre-kindergarten to Grade 12) in addition to controlling communicable illness and fostering health across the school population. School nurses support children in meeting goals of academic success and optimal wellness. "In successful school nursing practice, these goals weave seamlessly together to create a safety net and springboard for children to grow into healthy and successful citizens" (Wolfe, in Selekman, 2013, p. 26).

The school nurse is often likely to be the only healthcare provider in the educational setting. Other healthcare workers, such as occupational therapists or physical therapists, have specific caseloads within the school. The school nurse may be responsible for the entire student population in a given school, district, or identified region. The school nurse collaborates with other healthcare professionals to provide successful interventions that result in positive outcomes for the student. Today, communicable diseases are not the only health-related barriers to education. Some of the issues that school nurses must address include child abuse and or neglect; domestic and school violence; child and adolescent obesity and inactivity; mental health issues, including suicide and substance abuse; adolescent pregnancy and parenting; environmental health; physical and emotional disabilities and their consequences; chronic health needs; complex health conditions; and social determinants of health, such as family education, lack of health insurance coverage, homelessness, poverty, and more.

The healthcare consumer for the school nurse includes not only the student but also those influencing students, such as the family, school community, the larger surrounding community, aggregates within the school population, or the entire school population. Throughout this document, the term *student and school community* refers to the collective of school nursing clients. Nursing actions are directed to the student and school community. There are explicit times, however, when a school nursing standard refers directly to the student only; therefore, then, the term *student* is used.

Tenets of School Nursing Practice

1. *Caring and holistic health care are central to the practice of the school nurse.*

   As the health expert in the educational setting, the school nurse provides student-centered care, coordinating healing and health in a way that builds a relationship with the students and surrounding community. Using a holistic approach, the school nurse promotes an ongoing healthy environment that incorporates the physical, social, and emotional well-being of the student, the community, and society as a whole. The quality of caring is based on the relationship between the school nurse and the client: student, family, and community (Cowell, 2016b; Mason, Jones, Roy, & Sullivan, 2015).

2. *Nursing practice is individualized.*

   School nursing practice is respectful of diversity and cultural distinctions and the effect that these characteristics will have on providing health care. School nursing is individualized to meet the unique needs of the student and school community by coordinating a collaborative approach to comprehensive student-centered care. The student in the school community, defined as the individual student, and those influencing the student, such as the family, group, community, or population, is the focus of attention and to whom the school nurse is providing services as sanctioned by the state regulatory and governing bodies. While school nursing is population based, its unique purpose is to support each student for an optimal educational experience. School nurses use population outcomes such as attendance rates and immunization rates as well as individual health and educational outcomes such as adherence to prescribed regimens to evaluate effectiveness of their individualized care.

3. *RNs use the nursing process to plan and provide individualized care for students and the school community.*

   School nurses, using theoretical and evidence-based knowledge and the *Framework for 21st Century School Nursing Practice* (NASN, 2016c), advocate for and collaborate with students and school communities to evaluate and implement the principles and practices of health care that will optimize student success (Bultas & McLaughlin, 2013). As the healthcare professionals in educational settings, school nurses use critical thinking skills and the nursing process to address the individualized needs of their students and the populations they serve. School nurses advance the health of their populations through creating a "culture of health" within their school communities (Cowell, 2016a).

4. *Nurses coordinate care by establishing partnerships.*

   The school nurse establishes partnerships with persons, families, communities, support systems, primary healthcare providers, and other providers, using in-person and electronic communication methods, to reach a shared goal of delivering safe, quality health care for students and the school community. Collaborative, interprofessional team planning is based on recognition of the value and contributions, mutual trust, respect, open discussion, and shared decision-making of each discipline. Using the concept of holistic nursing, the school nurse coordinates and collaborates with all affiliates to promote a healthy environment that is conducive to student adaptation, self-management, self-advocacy, and educational success. Furthermore, as the primary healthcare providers employed in an educational setting, it is essential for school nurses to understand the overarching educational and organizational framework that guides their institutions and the roles they occupy within that environment (Wold and Selekman, 2013, p. 71).

5. *A strong link exists between the professional work environment and the ability of the school nurse to provide quality health care and achieve optimal outcomes.*

   School nurses have an ethical obligation to maintain and improve healthcare environments conducive to the provision of quality health care (ANA, 2015b). Elements of a healthy work environment have been extensively studied and demonstrate that the relationship between an environment free of negative, demoralizing, and unsafe conditions directly results in an enhanced quality of care that is without errors, workplace conflict, and moral stress. The school nurse must therefore commit to advocate to promote and sustain a healthy workplace.

The How of School Nursing

The "how" of school nursing practice is defined as the ways, means, methods, processes, and manner by which the school nurse practices professionally. To achieve the best health outcomes for student well-being, the "how" requires the school nurse to employ *evidence-based practice* as well as effective *interprofessional collaboration* within and across school communities.

ANA (2015b) noted that a chief component of the "how" of nursing is care coordination, which requires effective communication by all stakeholders. Therefore, the "how" of school nursing practice also encompasses communication skills to build and participate in effective teams and to communicate predictably and comprehensively using approaches such as informatics, electronic health records (EHRs), and systematic processes to reflect the manner in which school nurses respectfully care for students, their families, and the school community, leading to a *health-oriented system of care* (ANA, 2015b).

The ANA *Code of Ethics for Nurses with Interpretive Statements* (ANA, 2015a), the *NASN Code of Ethics for School Nurses* (NASN, 2016b), and ANA's *Nursing's Social Policy Statement* (ANA, 2010) guide the manner by which school nurses practice and advocate for the well-being and health of students and the school community. The "how" is further described by examining the science and art of school nursing and ways of practice that are described by the *Framework for 21st Century School Nursing Practice* and the Whole School, Whole Child, Whole Community model.

Science and Art of School Nursing

School nursing is both a science and an art. The *science* of school nursing provides evidence-based care dependent on research and critical thinking using the six steps of the nursing process. The *art* of school nursing combines caring, ethics, the personal knowledge and experiences of the nurse, interpersonal relationships, intuition, and the aesthetics of nursing to create holistic nursing practice and enhance the science of nursing (Chinn & Kramer, 2008). ANA (2015b) says that "the art of nursing embraces spirituality, healing, empathy, mutual respect, and compassion. . . . Healing is fostered by helping, listening, mentoring, coaching, teaching, exploring, being present, supporting, touching, intuition, service, cultural competence, tolerance, acceptance, nurturing, mutually creating, and conflict resolution" (p. 11). All of these combine to support the science and create the art of school nursing.

Science of School Nursing

The practice of school nursing is built upon sound theory, research, and consensus models of practice drawn from a large body of published work in nursing and school nursing, beginning with Nightingale (1860/1969). The actions of the school nurse focus on strengthening and facilitating students' educational and health outcomes through the application of theory and the implementation of evidence-based nursing care. Nursing actions are directed to the students and/or those influencing students such as the family, school community, the larger surrounding community, aggregates within the school population, or the entire school population.

The science of nursing relies on qualitative and quantitative evidence-based data as well as determining the school nurse impact on specific health outcomes. NASN has established a clear research agenda to support the science of school nursing, has engaged in a research-driven process to identify school nurse-sensitive indicators, and has begun a national data collection system to document school nursing practice and student outcomes (NASN, 2015). The NASN critical research priorities include the following:

- Determine the impact school nurse interventions have on students managing their chronic conditions (particularly *diabetes and asthma*).

- Determine the impact of school nurse interventions on *identified school-nurse-sensitive indicators* (attendance, seat time, early dismissal, health office visits, medication administration accuracy, and immunization rates).

- Conduct *cost–benefits analyses* of various interventions that can be used by the school nurse (care coordination, student safety, prevention services, and emergency room/911 visits).

- Evaluate *current models of school nurse practice* (i.e., RN per school or RN-supervising licensed practical nurses and unlicensed assistive personnel [UAPs] and/or covering multiple schools) and their impact on various outcomes (student safety, student physical and mental health, academics, access to care, and securing medical homes) (NASN, 2015).

The science of school nursing supports the school nurse as the liaison between the school, family, community healthcare providers, and the school-based or school-linked clinics. The school nurse is the healthcare expert within the school system and the leader in school health policy development, including identification of strategies to evaluate implementation of policies. As the healthcare expert, the school nurse provides leadership on wellness teams and implementation of the Whole School, Whole Child, Whole Community

Initiative (Centers for Disease Control and Prevention [CDC], 2015; ASCD & CDC, 2014) disaster preparedness teams, and the school health advisory councils. NASN (2016c) maintains that the practice of school nursing is unique because of the breadth of practice, including program management, and because the practice is set in a non-healthcare setting.

The school nurse must demonstrate competence in pediatric and adolescent health assessment, public health, community health, and adult and child mental health nursing. Competence in program management (including service delivery models), health promotion, family assessment, care coordination, communication, program planning, leadership, organization, and time management is essential. To be integrated into the school community, school nurses must be able to interpret the influence of health and education law on student health and learning, provide culturally congruent care, and be competent and comfortable functioning autonomously.

Art of School Nursing

School nurses practice the art of nursing. The art of school nursing is dependent on the culturally congruent care practiced by school nurses and based on complex interpersonal human relationships and a strong code of ethics.

The essence of the art of nursing is caring. With caring come courtesy, kindness, and respect for those provided nursing care. "A fundamental principle that underlies all nursing practice is respect for the inherent dignity, worth, unique attributes and human rights of all individuals" (ANA, 2015a, p. 1). Caring itself must be creative and intuitive for the greatest good for the students, families, and the school community and the school nurse. Each school nurse values every individual and group and works to meet unique cultural needs within legal and ethical parameters. School nursing standards describe competent nursing care, including the development of collaborative partnerships, the maintenance of interpersonal relationships, and careful inclusion and respect for diversity among others. School nurses create environments of trust, acceptance, and tolerance. School nurses demonstrate caring and culturally congruent practice by becoming part of the school community and through evaluating and addressing community needs. School nurses promote holistic care and wellness in students and communities, encourage appropriate independence in self-care and self-determination, and play an essential role in helping students navigate physical and emotional transitions within the educational system. School nurses model caring by their image, actions, and sensitivity to the individuals, families, groups, communities, and populations they serve.

The art of school nursing is emphasized in the Tenets of School Nursing Practice (see that section on pages 11 and 12) and further explicated by the new Standard 8: Culturally Congruent Practice and its associated competencies.

School nurses now have both a measure and accountability for provision of culturally competent care. Gently respecting cultural preferences and decisions while providing evidence-based practice with caring more clearly undergirds the goals of reduced health disparities and better outcomes. School nurses practice and model kindness, compassion, and courtesy for all in the school community to foster a healthy and safe environment.

The United States has many ethnicities that are the heritage of its citizenry. In a country where increased immigration is bringing together people of many backgrounds with associated diverse languages, health needs, and cultural practices, the school nurse must practice the art of nursing in a kind and compassionate manner. This requires consistent lifelong learning, an open mind, flexibility, and creativity. "Culturally competent nurses will increasingly serve as role models for novice clinicians, colleagues, and consumers, and as leaders of change" (Marion et al., 2016). School nurses, practicing the art and science of school nursing, have the opportunity to influence the cultural competence of the nation.

Framework for 21st Century School Nursing Practice

NASN developed the *Framework for 21st Century School Nursing Practice* to reflect current school nurse practice. Central to the framework is student-centered nursing care that occurs within the context of the students' families and the school community.

Framework Principles

Surrounding the student, family, and school community are the nonhierarchical, overlapping key principles of *Care Coordination, Leadership, Quality Improvement,* and *Community/Public Health.* These principles are surrounded by the fifth principle, *Standards of Practice,* which is the foundation for evidence-based, clinically competent, quality care. Each principle is further defined by practice components:

- *Care Coordination.* In daily practice, school nurses implement some or all of the following practice components of care coordination: case management, chronic disease management, collaborative communication, direct care, interdisciplinary teams, motivational interviewing/counseling, nursing delegation, student care plans, student-centered care, education, student self-empowerment, and transitional planning.

- *Leadership.* School nurses are well positioned in schools to lead in the development of school health policies, programs, and procedures for the provision of health services. The following competencies embrace the mindset of school nursing leadership: advocacy, change agent, education reform, funding and reimbursement, healthcare reform, lifelong learner, models of practice, technology, policy development and implementation, professionalism, and systems-level leadership.

- *Quality Improvement.* The principle of quality improvement describes an ongoing process that builds the critical evidence base to guide school nursing practice. Practice components involve continuous QI, documentation/data collection, evaluation, meaningful health and academic outcomes, performance appraisal, research, and uniform data set.

- *Community/Public Health.* School nurses utilize community/public health knowledge and skills to deliver nursing services within and across school populations. Components consist of access to care, cultural competency, disease prevention, environmental health, health education, health equity, Healthy People 2020 objectives, health promotion, outreach, population-based care, risk reduction, screening/referral/follow-up, social determinants of health, and surveillance.

- *Standards of Practice.* The Standards of Practice are critical to direct and lead all principles of the framework. Standards of practice components include clinical competence, clinical guidelines, code of ethics, critical thinking, evidence-based practice, NASN position statements, nurse practice acts, and scope and standards of practice documents.

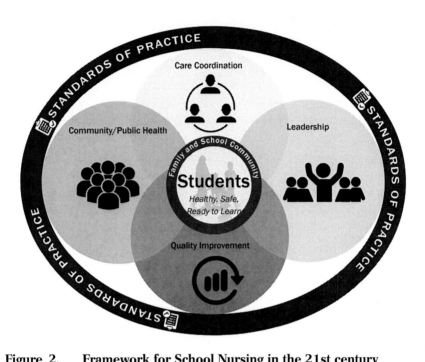

Figure 2. **Framework for School Nursing in the 21st century (NASN, 2015).**

Within the how of school nursing, the *Framework for 21st Century School Nursing Practice* (Figure 2) is aligned with the Whole School, Whole Community, Whole Child (WSCC) model to guide the practice of school nursing.

Whole School, Whole Community, Whole Child

The Centers for Disease Control and Prevention (CDC) and the ASCD revised the more narrowly defined coordinated school health approach to a broader Whole School, Whole Community, Whole Child (WSCC) model (ASCD & CDC, 2015; Lewellen et al., 2014).

The tenets of the WSCC approach are for each student to

- Enter school healthy and learn to practice a healthy lifestyle.
- Learn in an environment that is physically and emotionally safe for students and adults.
- Be actively engaged in learning and connected to the school and broader community.

- Have access to personalized learning that is supported by qualified, caring adults.
- Be challenged academically and prepared for success in college, career, and life ready to participate in a global environment.

To promote greater alignment between health and educational outcomes, the WSCC model includes Health Education; Nutrition Environment and Services; Employee Wellness; Social and Emotional School Climate; Physical Environment; Health Services; Counseling, Psychological, and Social Services; Community Involvement; Family Engagement; and Physical Education and Physical Activity (http://www.cdc.gov/healthyschools/wscc/components.htm):

- *Health Education.* Formal, structured health education consists of a combination of planned, developmentally appropriate learning experiences that provide knowledge and skills that students need to make quality health decisions.
- *Nutrition Environment and Services.* The school nutrition environment provides students with opportunities to learn about and practice healthy eating through available foods and beverages, nutrition education, and messages about food in the cafeteria and throughout the school campus.
- *Employee Wellness.* Fostering school employees' good health protects school staff and, by doing so, helps to support student outcomes of wellness and academic success.
- *Social and Emotional School Climate.* The social and emotional climate of a school can impact student engagement in school activities, relationships with other students, staff, family, and community; and academic performance.
- *Physical Environment.* The physical school environment encompasses the school building and its contents, the land on which the school is located, and the area surrounding it.
- *Health Services.* Health services actively connect school staff, students, families, communities, and healthcare providers to promote the health care of students and a healthy and safe school environment.
- *Counseling, Psychological, and Social Services.* These prevention and intervention services support the mental, behavioral, and social-emotional health of students and promote success in the learning process.

- *Community Involvement.* Community groups, organizations, and local businesses create partnerships with schools, share resources, and volunteer to support student learning, development, and health-related activities.

- *Family Engagement.* Families and school staff work together to support and improve the learning, development, and health of students.

- *Physical Education and Physical Activity.* Physical education provides cognitive content and instruction designed to develop motor skills, knowledge, and behaviors for healthy active living, physical fitness, sportsmanship, self-efficacy, and emotional intelligence.

The *Framework for 21st Century Nursing Practice* and the WSCC model clearly shape the art and science of school nursing practice.

Where Does School Nursing Occur? School Nursing Settings

"Nursing occurs in any environment where there is a healthcare consumer in need of care, information, or advocacy" (ANA, 2015b, p. 19). School nurses provide care in the school environment and work setting, considering acuity of student needs and the unique attributes of the student body and surrounding community, including the social determinants of health.

In the realm of school health, school nurses practice within the educational environment. Although school nurses are typically employed by local school districts or school boards, other entities such as public health agencies, colleges, hospitals, private health corporations, private school corporations, religious entities, and tribal agencies may also be the employer. School nursing usually happens in a school building and/or district; however, with its foundation in public health, school nursing practice extends into communities. School nursing is practiced at juvenile justice centers, alternative treatment centers, hospital schools, preschools, Magnet and charter schools, private and parochial schools, Department of Defense schools, and schools on college campuses. Some school nurses make home visits, and in some states, school nurses provide services to families with infants and toddlers with disabilities exclusively within their homes. Advocacy is fundamental to school nursing practice in all settings (ANA, 2015b).

On the individual level, school nurses interact with students, school staff, families, primary healthcare providers, and community agencies. As student health and social needs have changed, culturally congruent practice has gained increased importance to effectively continue these collaborations. Now, for the school nurse to support and meet the needs of a global society, the acquisition of cultural skills by the school nurse is essential. Providing effective management of chronic conditions, promoting the maintenance of health and the prevention of disease, and furnishing an environment of caring and safety require an ongoing engagement of culturally competent lifelong learning (Carr & Knutson, 2015).

By fostering interpersonal relationships, school nurses provide support, information, and access to resources for students and their families. School nurses are encouraged to serve on committees and boards within their schools, communities, state, and nation that pertain to student health and success. This participation improves the health of the community, increases access to resources, and promotes networking partnerships. By practicing culturally congruent student-centered nursing care, the school nurse becomes the voice for the students, their families, and the school community as a whole.

Through advocacy, school nurses promote student health. At the school district level, the school nurse should be involved with school policies concerning the delivery of health services, including, but not limited to, health service staffing based on student acuity and needs, nursing delegation, medications, infection control, injury management, automated external defibrillation (AED) programs, and school staff training. At the community level, the school nurse advocates for services for students, such as safe environments, adequate shelter, and accessible health services (physical, mental, and dental) along with employment and recreational opportunities. On a state and national level, school nurses advocate for legislation to improve students' lives. This may include educational funding, equity in education, safe schools, appropriate health service staffing, and government policies that ensure that all students have adequate housing, food, and educational opportunities to succeed at school.

School nurses advocate for health accommodations that will enable a student to achieve greater success at school. Along with advocating for students, school nurses promote the school nurse specialty. With school budget cuts comes the threat that many school nursing positions may be eliminated or replaced with less qualified individuals who are unsupervised by registered professional nurses. When students with increasingly complex health needs enter the general school population, delegation of care *may* be necessary, but only after careful determination is made by a registered professional nurse (NASN, 2014a). Delegation of care can only occur in compliance with state nurse practice acts and accompanying local and state laws and regulations.

School-Based Health Centers and Wellness Centers

Some schools have primary care clinics located in schools. School-based health centers (SBHCs) or wellness centers were developed in the 1970s to provide healthcare services to students who could not afford or easily access primary health care. School nurses provide assessment and referral for individual students with specific needs to center staff for appropriate services. Primary care for students with parent permission, when required, at the centers may include medical, dental, nutrition, social, emotional, and mental health services, while school nurses provide support as leaders in the school community, providing oversight for the health and safety of the students through school health policies and programs. School nurses and SBHC staff often work in collaboration to develop policies, collect data, and evaluate processes to improve health outcomes for students and the communities they serve (NASN, 2016d). It is important to note that "one does not replace the other" (NASN, 2016d), meaning SBHCs cannot replace the need for or expertise of the school nurse. However, school nurses and staff from the SBHCs, including APRNs, work together in a collaborative relationship to meet the healthcare needs of the students and school community.

Other Environments in School Nurse Practice

School nursing can also be responsible for the health and safety of *all students, including those students with special needs*, when they participate in activities outside of the classroom and boundaries of the school building.

- *Playground*: Ensuring safe, age-appropriate, well-maintained playground equipment with adequate supervision will increase safety for children. Development of a playground safety plan by the school nurse is vital for the prevention of student injuries (Olsen, Hudson, & Thompson, 2008).

- *Bus transportation*: Students with special needs, especially those with associated respiratory or mobility issues, must have transportation safety needs included in their healthcare plans and emergency plans. Collaboration with transportation officials can help to provide healthy outcomes for students. Additionally, the environment is a concern in school bus transportation. The high prevalence of asthma in children requires school nurses to ensure implementation of clean air policies, including limiting children's exposure to school bus diesel emissions and other air pollutants. School nurses can advocate for a reduction in those emissions by promoting idle free zones (Mazer, Jacobson Vann, Lamanna, & Davison, 2014).

- *Field trips*: Students' educational experiences can be enhanced by field trips. When the student has special healthcare needs, planning for positive experiences requires coordination by the school nurse, primary healthcare provider, family, and staff. Extra attention must be paid to state nurse practice act issues involving interstate school trips (Erwin, Clark, & Mercer, 2014).

- *Before- and after-school programs, athletic programs, and extracurricular activities*: When school nurses and athletic trainers collaborate, the well-being and safety of the student, family, and community are improved. By sharing health and injury prevention plans, communication is enhanced among school employees to ensure that students with health concerns can participate and injuries can be prevented (Rains & Robinson, 2012). Communication with before- and after-school care program staff is also necessary for student healthcare coordination and injury prevention.

Healthy Work Environments for School Nursing

The importance of a healthy work environment emerged as a direct result of two publications: the IOM report *To Err Is Human: Building a Safer Health System* (IOM, 1999) and *Crossing the Quality Chasm* (IOM, 2001). A consequence of these reports resulted in the formation of the Quality and Safety Education for Nurses (QSEN) (Dolansky & Moore, 2013). Funded by the Robert Wood Johnson Foundation, this 2005 QSEN initiative highlighted the essential components necessary to deliver quality, safe care in a healthy work environment. With the focus on key aspects that support optimal health and safety, nurses and other healthcare professionals must be mindful of what is necessary to achieve these in the area of clinical practice:

- Patient-centered care
- Teamwork and collaboration
- Evidence-based practice
- Quality improvement
- Safety
- Informatics (Rosenblum & Sprague-McRae, 2014).

The American Association of Critical-Care Nurses criteria for healthy work environments that establish and maintain an interdependent, healthy work environment, include six standards and require all nurses to

- Be proficient in skilled communication,
- Foster true collaboration with partners,
- Be effective decision-makers in policy and in leading organizations,
- Ensure appropriate staffing,

- Foster recognition of self and others, and

- Embrace the role of a leader in creating and sustaining a healthy work environment (Barden, Cassidy, & Cardin, 2016, p. 10).

These principles of a healthy employment environment suitably apply to nurses who work as health professionals in an educational setting. In this environment, the school nurse is required to initiate and maintain collaboration at an interprofessional level; to communicate the important contributions of nursing to the academic success of students; and to assume leadership roles in student assistance teams, wellness committees, and staff health promotion policies and activities. To facilitate this, it is essential that the school nurse use continuing education resources to remain current in the latest evidence-based research pertaining to school health (Rosenblum & Sprague-McRae, 2014).

In addition, evidence demonstrates that negative, demoralizing, and unsafe conditions in the workplace, emanating from a physically or psychologically unhealthy environment, contribute to nursing errors, ineffective delivery of care, and conflict and stress among health or other professionals and those they serve. Hostile and/or violent working conditions can impact the school environment and school nurse retention (ANA, 2015b; Castronovo, Pullizzi, & Evans, 2016; Cowell, 2016b). The school nurse is responsible for providing and advocating for a continuous healthy work environment in the school setting to promote a "culture of safety" (ANA, 2015b, p. 21).

Workloads and Acuity

Workloads and their acuity are critical components of a healthy work environment for school nurses. Many times, workloads assigned to individual school nurses are unrealistic and unmanageable. As the complexity of the health and socioeconomic needs of students has increased, so has the need to expand the number of school nurses necessary to provide care coordination necessary to facilitate positive student health and academic achievement (McClanahan & Weismuller, 2015). In 2016, The American Academy of Pediatrics (2016) called for a minimum of one full-time RN in every school. NASN (2016e) also states that all students should have access to a school nurse all day, every day. Recommendations for simple nurse to student ratios do not always accurately reflect the health services needed; therefore, NASN recommends that acuity, complex needs of students, and social determinants of health must also be considered when evaluating staffing patterns (NASN, 2015).

Another component of optimal staffing that benefits nurses and consumers is a team-based approach. The ANA (2015b) notes that "contemporary staffing models should include elements that support team-based care which has been identified as a highly effective model that promotes safe, effective and efficient care" (p. 23). School nurses are members of interprofessional school teams that collaborate to address the learning needs of students in a healthy and safe school environment.

When School Nursing Occurs

School nursing occurs whenever there is a need to provide specialized nursing that advances the well-being, academic success, and lifelong achievement of the student population. In partnership with the student, family, school staff, and other healthcare providers, the school nurse is able to influence actual and potential health problems. Using knowledge, research, and evidence-based practice, the school nurse translates prevailing recommendations into clinical practice, with the goal of keeping students safe, healthy, and ready to learn.

School settings commonly reflect a culturally and socially diverse student population. It is essential, therefore, that the school nurse is in a position to provide culturally competent care by understanding the values, beliefs, and practices of students and their families. School-aged children spend a signif-icant part of the day away from their families. Thus, it is important for the school nurse to be culturally aware and effectively communicate within mul-tiple population groups.

Students with Special Needs

The school nurse practices in an environment that has changed dramatically since the early 20th century. The Individuals with Disabilities Education Act of 1975 (with several subsequent revisions), Section 504 of the Rehabilitation Act of 1973, the Americans with Disabilities Act of 1990, and the ensu-ing American with Disabilities Amendment Act of 2008 have contributed to removing barriers that have hindered students' access to education and bring greater clarification to the definition of a disability (Sampson & Galemore, 2012). Education regulations and legislative directives heighten the complexity of decision-making and practice, such as those of the Family Education Rights and Privacy Act (FERPA) of 1974 and do not resuscitate (DNR) or do not attempt resuscitation (DNAR) orders issued for the school setting. It is incum-bent upon the school nurse to become familiar with their state and district laws (Zacharski et al., 2013). The privacy restrictions to medical information by the Health Information Portability and Accountability Act (HIPAA) of 1996 present an ongoing challenge to school nurses who need information about student healthcare needs for the provision of adequate care at school. Electronic health records (EHRs) have improved communication between nurses and among providers (Radis, Updegrove, Somsel, & Crowley, 2016).

A unique role for the nurse in the school is the provision of nursing services to children with unique learning and physical abilities. These include, but are not limited to, physical, behavioral, and emotional variances; specific conditions including acute or chronic illnesses; and speech and learning delays and disorders. The school nurse, often in collaboration with interprofessional teams, develops healthcare plans unique to the school setting. Among these are the following: the Individualized Healthcare Plan (IHP), Individualized Education Plan or Program (IEP), and the Section 504 Plan (Galemore & Sheetz, 2015). Transition plans for adolescent-aged students in special education may include healthcare transition plans. Many states and school district regulations or procedures include plans in addition to, or instead of, these—for example, the Emergency Care Plan or Emergency Action Plan and crisis management or disaster management plans. In all cases, when a student is in need of accommodation for positive educational and life outcomes, it is vital that the school nurse play a leadership role in advocacy for the student in developing and implementing the plan most suited to the student's needs.

Environmental Health

Ongoing environmental health efforts continue some of the earliest foci of school nursing. Lillian Wald, who was a pioneer public health nurse and an early leader in school nursing, followed the advice of Florence Nightingale, who demonstrated that cleanliness in the environment affected the health of patients and suggested that all nurses practice cleanliness (Nightingale, 1860/1969). The huge numbers of people who spend their days in schools suggest that the cleanliness of the school environment can affect the health of many Americans. In fall 2016, the U.S. Department of Education estimated that 50.4 million students and 3.1 million teachers were in public schools and 5.2 million students and 0.4 million teachers were studying in private schools in the United States (National Center for Education Statistics, 2016). Support staff, potentially in the millions, were not included in the data.

Environmental health, a branch of public health, is concerned with all aspects of the natural and built environment. NASN's (2014b) interpretation of the 2011 World Health Organization report on the environment and potential effects on health suggests that the school nurse has the educational and clinical background required to understand the issues of environmental health in the school setting and is in a prime position to advocate for a sustainable healthy school environment.

Today's school environment can be filled with many types of environmental pollutants (Mazer et al., 2013) and communicable and infectious agents that can affect the health and welfare of students and others in the school community (Luthy, Houle, Beckstrand, Macintosh, & Larkin, 2013). The school nurse, as the health expert in the school, can help to mitigate or eliminate environmental pollutants and pathogenic organisms in the school setting. Finally, the school nurse contributes to safeguarding the environment by participating in the development and implementation of emergency and disaster preparedness plans.

Professional School Nurses: The Who of School Nursing

Members of the school nursing specialty include registered nurses (RNs), graduate-level-prepared registered nurses, and advanced practice registered nurses who have been educated, titled, and maintain active licensure to practice. Educational preparation of school nurses varies. Because of the broad scope of the specialty practice and the complexity of issues addressed within a school community setting by the school nurse requiring advanced skills, which include the ability to practice independently, supervise others, and delegate care, NASN recommends that the minimal educational preparation for a school nurse be a BSN degree from an accredited college or university, as well as state certification in those states requiring or recommending state school nurse licensure/certification. Specialty certification for nurses with a BSN or higher education improves patient outcomes, and baccalaureate-educated nurses with specialty certification have the potential to improve the quality of care (Kendall-Gallagher, Aiken, Sloane, Douglas, & Cimotti, 2011; NASN, 2016a).

Meeting the BSN degree or state certification credentials is strongly encouraged for those school nurses who may have entered the field without these recommended credentials. All school nurses must seek professional development and continuing education to increase critical thinking skills and professional judgment as well as to maintain competence in their role. NASN also recommends that school nurses demonstrate knowledge of school nursing by acquiring school nursing specialty certification from the National Board for Certification of School Nurses (NBCSN). The baccalaureate degree is the minimum level of education required for applicants for the national school nurse certification examination. The awarded National Certified School Nurse credential must be renewed every 5 years through professional development or reexamination. Additionally, some school nurses may hold other specialty certifications, such as a public health nursing certification.

Given their preparation and expertise, some school nurses practice as school nurse specialists, such as school nurse consultants, school nurse supervisors and administrators, lead nurses or school health team leaders, school nurses with advanced clinical preparation, and in other specialty roles. School nurses are in lead roles within school districts, charter, private and parochial schools, regions and counties, and at the state level. Some have pursued advanced academic studies to prepare for specialization in practice.

Graduate-Level-Prepared School Nurses

Graduate-level-prepared school nurses are prepared at the master's or doctoral educational level (e.g., MSN, PhD, EdD, DNSc, or DNP); have advanced knowledge, skills, abilities, and judgment; function in an advanced level as designated by elements of the nurse's position; and are not required to have additional regulatory oversight (ANA, 2015b). Their advanced education may be in school nursing, administration, education, case management, nursing informatics, public health, research, or other health and nursing areas of study. In graduate programs of study, nurses advance their knowledge and skills in clinical areas related to the programs, as well as in research.

The practice of the graduate-level-prepared school nurse focuses on four concepts:

- *Populations.* Graduate-level-prepared school nurses are leaders in population assessment, drawing on multiple data sources to synthesize population needs. Many graduate-level-prepared school nurses have combined job descriptions and responsibilities that include provision of direct care to students as well as responsibilities for leading population-level care.

- *Systems.* Graduate-level-prepared school nurses work in multiple sectors and with multiple disciplines serving the student and school community. They work at systems levels and are experts in communications that maximize interactions throughout systems.

- *Complexity.* Graduate-level-prepared school nurses are skilled at managing and solving complex, multilevel, and simultaneously occurring problems and issues.

- *Growth of the specialty.* Graduate-level-prepared school nurses assume leadership positions to actively engage in defining, articulating the direction, and advancing the specialty of school nursing. They also evaluate, conduct, and apply evidence-based research to advance the specialty of and engage in the development of standards and guidelines for school nursing practice.

A graduate-level-prepared school nurse is expected to comply with the standards of practice and professional performance for school nursing, the associated competencies for all school nurses, and the additional competencies for a graduate-level-prepared school nurse. Resources such as *Nursing Administration: Scope and Standards of Practice* (ANA, 2016) or *Public Health Nursing: Scope and Standards of Practice, 2nd Edition* (ANA, 2013) may provide additional direction.

Advanced Practice Registered Nurses

Advanced practice registered nurses are those

- Who have completed an accredited graduate-level education program preparing the nurse for four recognized roles, including certified nurse practitioner (CNP), clinical nurse specialist (CNS), certified nurse midwife (CNM), or certified registered nurse anesthetist (CRNA);

- Who have passed a national certification examination that measures APRN, role, and population-focused competencies and maintain competence as evidenced by recertification through the national certification program;

- Who have acquired advanced clinical knowledge and skills preparing the nurse to provide direct care to patients, as well as a component of indirect care;

- Whose practices build on the competencies of RNs by demonstrating a greater depth and breadth of knowledge, a greater synthesis of data, increased complexity of skills and interventions, and a greater role autonomy;

- Who are educationally prepared to assume responsibility and accountability for health promotion and/or maintenance as well as the assessment, diagnosis, and management of patient problems, which includes the use of and prescription of pharmacologic and nonpharmacologic interventions;

- Who have clinical experience of sufficient depth and breadth to reflect the intended license; and

- Who have obtained a license to practice as an APRN in one of four APRN roles: CRNA, CNM, CNS, or CNP (ANA, 2015b, pp. 2–3).

Some school nurses may meet the standards identified for APRNs as a result of their education, experience, skill, and authority to practice granted by their state licensing board. In schools, APRNs may be nurse practitioners, CNPs, or both. APRNs are often part of an enhanced school services team, a school-based health center, or a wellness center that provides direct diagnostic and treatment care to students.

An APRN working in a combined APRN and school nurse role is expected to comply with the standards of practice and professional performance and associated competencies for all school nurses, the competencies for graduate-level-prepared school nurses, and the additional competencies for an APRN. The APRN role in the school may be limited by job description or agency policy.

In addition to requirements for APRNs listed in the Consensus Model for APRN Regulation: Licensure, Accreditation, Certification, and Education (APRN Joint Dialog Group, 2008), the following organizations and resources address standards and competencies for advanced practice roles school nurses might hold:

- American Association of Nurse Practitioners: *Standards of Practice for Nurse Practitioners* (2013)
- American Nurses Credentialing Center (http://www.nursecredential ing.org)
- National Organization of Nurse Practitioner Faculties: *Domains and Core Competencies of Nurse Practitioner Practice* (2012)
- *Population-Focused Nurse Practitioner Competencies: Family/Across the Lifespan, Neonatal, Pediatric Acute Care, Pediatric Primary Care, Psychiatric Mental Health, and Women's Health/Gender-Specific* (Population Focused Competencies Task Force, 2013)
- National Association of Clinical Nurse Specialists

Statistics of the Profession

A Health Resources and Services Administration (HRSA) analysis indicates that 61,323 RNs work in elementary and secondary schools (HRSA 2013: *The US Nursing Workforce: Trends in Supply and Education*). In addition, the DoDEA reports that 168 school nurses serve students and families in DoDEA schools for children of the military in 2015–2016 (R. Shepherd, personal e-mail communication with DoDEA, July 2016).

Results of the 2015 NASN School Nurse Survey, which targeted all school nurses and elicited responses from members and nonmembers of the organization, indicate that nearly half (45.3%) of 7,901 respondents had a bachelor's degree in nursing (BSN), 15% had an associate's degree (ADN), 11.5% had a master's degree in nursing (MS/MSN), and 0.3% held a doctorate in nursing. Nonnursing degrees held by school nurses included bachelor's degree in other fields (4.7%), master's degree in education (5.2%), master's degree in other field (4.4%), master's in public health (MPH) (0.8%), and doctorates in other field (0.3%). Almost 23% (22.7%) of respondents were nationally certified by the National Board for the Certification of School Nurses. Fifty-five percent of respondents held state school nurse certification. Finally, 36.2% of the school nurses reported being evaluated by an RN.

The survey indicated that 83% of school nurses were employed by a public school district, where they worked in an average of three buildings with an average of 924 to 1,072 students. Five percent of respondents worked for private/parochial/boarding schools, 4% for public health departments, and 1% for hospital/HMO/health systems (NASN, 2015, School Nurse Survey).

Professional Competence in School Nursing Practice

The school community has a right to expect school nurses to demonstrate professional competence throughout their careers. The school nurse is individually responsible and accountable for maintaining professional competence. Beyond individual responsibility, NASN and ANA further believe that it is the nursing profession's responsibility to shape and guide any process for assuring nurse competence. Regulatory agencies define minimal standards for regulation of nursing practice to protect the public. Finally, the employer is responsible and accountable to provide a practice environment conducive to competent school nursing practice. Therefore, assurance of competence is the shared responsibility of the profession, individual school nurses, professional organizations, credentialing and certification entities, regulatory agencies, employers, and other key stakeholders (adapted from ANA, 2015b, p. 43).

NASN and ANA believe that, in the practice of nursing, competence can be defined, measured, and evaluated. No single evaluation method or tool can guarantee competence. Competence is situational and dynamic; it is both an outcome and an ongoing process. Context determines what competencies are necessary.

A number of terms and concepts are central to the discussion of the ongoing demonstration of competence:

- An individual who demonstrates competence is performing at an expected level.

- A *competency* is an expected level of performance that integrates knowledge, skills, abilities, and judgment.

- The integration of knowledge, skills, abilities, and judgment occurs in formal, informal, and reflective learning experiences.

- Knowledge encompasses critical thinking, understanding of science and humanities, use of professional standards of practice, and insights gained from context, practical experiences, personal capabilities, and leadership performance.

- Skills include psychomotor, communication, interpersonal, and diagnostic skills.

- Ability is the capacity to act effectively. It requires listening, integrity, knowledge of one's strengths and weaknesses, positive self-regard, emotional intelligence, and openness to feedback.

- Judgment includes critical thinking, problem solving, ethical reasoning, and decision-making (ANA, 2015b, p. 44).

Types of learning associated with the development of competency include formal learning, informal learning, and reflective learning. Formal learning most often occurs in structured, academic, and professional development practice environments, while informal learning can be described as experiential insights gained from work, community, home, and other settings. The recurrent, thoughtful, personal self-assessment, analysis, and synthesis of strengths and opportunities for improvement constitute reflective learning. Such insights should lead to the creation of a specific plan for professional development and may become part of a school nurse's professional portfolio (ANA, 2015b).

School nurses are influenced by the nature of the practice situation, which includes consideration of the setting; resources; and the individual, family, group, community, or population. Practice situations can either enhance or detract from the school nurse's ability to provide quality care. The school nurse influences factors that facilitate and enhance competent practice and seeks to deal with barriers that constrain competent practice. The expected level of performance reflects variability depending on the school nursing practice situation and the selected practice framework or model.

The ability to perform at the expected level requires a process of lifelong learning. School nurses must continually reassess their competencies and identify needs for additional knowledge, skills, personal growth, and integrative learning experiences (adapted from ANA, 2015b, p. 44).

Evaluating Competence

Competence in school nursing practice must be evaluated by the individual nurse (self-assessment), school nurse peers, and nurses in the roles of supervisor, coach, or mentor or preceptor. In addition, other aspects of performance not exclusive to the practice of nursing (e.g., interpersonal and communication skills, team collaboration and networking, and classroom teaching) may be evaluated by professional colleagues, administrators, and others. Evaluation of competence involves using tools to capture objective and subjective data about the individual's knowledge and actual performance. Those tools must be appropriate for the specific school nursing situation and the desired outcome of the competence evaluation. Such tools and methods include, but are not limited to, direct observation, records, portfolios, demonstrations, skills lab, performance evaluation, peer review, certification, credentialing, privileging, simulation exercises, computer-simulated and virtual reality testing, targeted continuing education with outcomes measurement, employer skills validation, and practice evaluations. However, no single evaluation tool or method can guarantee competence (ANA, 2015b).

The Why of School Nursing
Ethical Considerations in School Nursing

The practice of school nursing requires vigilant attention to ethics. The school nurse is an advocate for students, families, and school communities. The school nurse provides age-appropriate and culturally congruent care to students and the school community. The school nurse promotes active, informed participation in health decisions; respects the individual's right to be treated with dignity; and understands the ethical and legal issues surrounding an individual's right to privacy and confidentiality. The school nurse treats all members of the school community equally, regardless of race, gender, social or economic status, culture, age, sexual orientation, disability, or religion.

The school nurse maintains the highest level of competence by enhancing professional knowledge and skills; collaborating with peers, other health professionals, and community agencies; and adhering to *Nursing's Social Policy Statement: The Essence of the Profession* (ANA, 2010), *Code of Ethics for Nurses with Interpretive Statements* (ANA, 2015a), *Code of Ethics with Interpretive Statements for the School Nurse* (NASN, 2016b), and this document, *School Nursing: Scope and Standards of Practice, Third Edition.* School nurses participate in efforts to advance and use the standards of practice, expand the body of school nursing knowledge through nursing research, and improve conditions of the workplace environment. School nurses are expected to self-regulate as they are responsible to themselves and others for the quality of their practices. The school nurse is autonomous and must engage in personal accountability for quality assurance.

The Code of Ethics for Nurses in School Nursing Practice

The following provisions from *Code of Ethics for Nurses with Interpretive Statements* (ANA, 2015a) are printed without the interpretive statements and are explored characterizing the specialty of school nursing.

Provision 1. The nurse practices with compassion and respect for the inherent dignity, worth, and unique attributes of every person.

Key characteristics of this provision for the school nurse include respecting human dignity; establishing relationships with the student, parents, and staff; respecting the student's health status; recognizing right to self-determination; and maintaining professional, respectful, and caring relationships.

Compassion is a value inherent in the role of school nursing. School nurses respect the dignity and unique attributes of students, staff, and parents. School nurses understand the variable health status of each student. School nurses recognize the necessity to maintain clear boundaries while establishing caring and respectful relationships with the student, staff, and parent. School nurses serve all students in their communities encompassing a wide range of characteristics, for example, race and ethnicity, children with special health or educational needs, and immigrant students. With compassion and respect, they work closely with school staff, healthcare providers, families, and their communities to identify and address the individual needs of the students.

***Provision 2.* The nurse's primary commitment is to the patient, whether an individual, family, group, community, or population.**

Key characteristics of this provision for the school nurse include prioritizing student health and emotional need, avoiding conflicts of interest, collaborating with school staff and local community, and establishing professional boundaries regarding the school environment.

School nurses interpret and explain students' health needs to the education team, helping them to understand the significance and possible impact on academic achievement. As well, school nurses assist the community to understand students' needs for professional nursing services within the educational environment. When there are issues regarding student care, as an example, a student's refusal of a specific medication or treatment, the school nurse is committed to supporting the student's well-informed, intentional, and careful decision. This can sometimes lead to conflict. However, the school nurse's primary commitment is to the student, and therefore to work with the student and family to come to a safe and appropriate resolution.

***Provision 3.* The nurse promotes, advocates for, and protects the rights, health, and safety of the patient.**

Key characteristics of this provision for the school nurse include protection of the rights of privacy and confidentiality, protection of students and vulnerable populations in research, adherence to performance standards and review mechanisms, maintenance of policies that promote a culture of safety, acting on questionable practice in self or others, and protection of students if there is possible impaired practice within the educational setting.

In collaboration with stakeholders, school nurses develop, implement, and evaluate individual plans of care that can include educational accommodations based on identified health needs of students to promote their success. For students with life-threatening health conditions, the school nurse collaborates with the parents and healthcare providers to ensure that emergency medications are available at school and all appropriate staff are trained to support the child in an emergency situation.

Provision 4. **The nurse has authority, accountability, and responsibility for nursing practice; makes decisions; and takes action consistent with the obligation to promote health and to provide optimal care.**

Key characteristics of this provision for the school nurse include accountability for nursing judgment; decisions and actions, responsibility for nursing judgment decisions and actions; and assignments and delegation of nursing activities or tasks, including supervision of unlicensed assistive personnel (when legally appropriate).

As the primary healthcare provider in the school setting, the school nurse is in an ideal position to identify, instruct, and monitor personnel to provide valuable assistance in meeting the healthcare needs of students. More students are diagnosed with chronic health conditions such as asthma, diabetes, and life-threatening allergies. In order to provide optimal care for these students so they may participate in all school events—particularly off-campus events—the school nurse has the responsibility to ensure that a qualified UAP member is available to accompany these students on their trip and, within the guidelines of the student's healthcare plan, safely administer care when necessary.

Provision 5. **The nurse owes the same duty to self as to others, including the responsibility to promote health and safety, preserve wholeness of character and integrity, maintain competence, and continue personal and professional growth.**

Key characteristics of this provision for the school nurse include respect to self and others; promotion of personal health, safety, and well-being; preservation of wholeness of character; preservation of integrity; maintenance of competence; and continuation of professional and personal growth.

In many instances, the school nurse reports to an administrator with a background in education, rather than a healthcare supervisor. The collaboration between administrators and school nurses, at times, can result in ethical dilemmas for the nurse. One such situation is being asked to delegate a nursing activity that may be unsafe for the child. By being aware of emerging child health issues, knowing the state nurse practice acts, implementing the latest evidence-based practice in the health office, and having access to peer-reviewed journals relating to current trends in child and school health, a school nurse is better equipped to demonstrate the knowledge and leadership qualities that are brought to promote the health and safety of the entire school community. Additionally, due to the independent nature of their roles, school nurses need to actively engage in self-care skills that promote the "healthy" nurse, such as walking, gardening, pleasure reading, and other holistic strategies.

Provision 6. **The nurse, through individual and collective effort, establishes, maintains, and improves the ethical environment of the work setting and conditions of employment that are conducive to safe, quality health care.**

Key characteristics of this provision for the school nurse include moral virtue, ethical obligation, and responsibility to the work environment in order to support student learning.

Working with other professionals in the school community, school nurses can address inequities such as unhealthy indoor air quality, mold in schools, and unsafe playgrounds to promote healthy environments. School nurses also address a healthy social environment and ensure that all students feel safe and supported regardless of their gender, race, sexual orientation, or abilities.

Provision 7. **The nurse, in all roles and settings, advances the profession through research and scholarly inquiry, professional standards development, and the generation of both nursing and health policy.**

Key characteristics of this provision for the school nurse include contribution through research and scholarly inquiry; contribution through developing, maintaining, and implementing professional practice standards; and contribution through policy development.

Through quality improvement and best practices, school nurses can advocate for student health services based on appropriate workload for the student population. If the needs of the students, such as chronic health concerns, medication management, and medical treatments, are significant, additional health services may be justified. School nurses also advance their professional through implementation of clinical guidelines and evidence-based practice tools offered by the National Association of School Nurses.

Provision 8. **The nurse collaborates with other health professionals and the public to protect human rights, promote health diplomacy, and reduce health disparities.**

Key characteristics of this provision for the school nurse include health as a universal right; collaboration for health, human rights, and health diplomacy; obligation to advance health and human rights and reduce disparities; and collaboration for human rights in complex, extreme, or extraordinary practice settings.

The 21st century school nurse model promotes care coordination with students' healthcare providers. If a student has a chronic health condition, such as asthma, the school nurse can collaborate with the family and healthcare provider to ensure that the student has health insurance and access to appropriate care, such as asthma specialists. On a more global level, the school nurse also advocates for clean, safe, affordable housing free of environmental triggers, such as mold, for our students with asthma and safe, uncontaminated water—free of lead—such as the work of school nurses in Flint, Michigan.

Provision 9. The profession of nursing, collectively through its professional organizations, must articulate nursing values, maintain the integrity of the profession, and integrate principles of social justice into nursing and health policy.

Key characteristics of this provision for the school nurse include participation in professional nursing associations, promotion of awareness of adherence to the code of ethics for nurses, and participation in social justice activities statewide, nationally, and globally.

Membership in professional organizations, such as NASN, allows the school nurse to connect to the larger community of school nurses for education and sharing resources. National certification from the National Board for Certification of School Nurses indicates competence in school nurse practice. Both membership and certification are encouraged for the professional school nurse to maintain a high level of ethics to be leaders in school nursing and to advocate for the needs of students.

Ethical Challenges in School Nursing

The degree to which the total school community supports school nursing practice affects the delivery of nursing care and, hence, the ethical nature of that care. Inadequate staffing may contribute to the ineffective delivery of care, compromise staff and student wellness, and contribute to conflict and stress among school nursing professionals. School nurses may face ethical challenges when responding to the increased demands of caring for children with complex healthcare needs. Often, those children consume much of the school nurse's time. School nurses may struggle with balancing the needs of children with complex healthcare needs while assuring that the general school population needs are met. Additionally, the geographic distance between schools may be such that nurses spend considerable time traveling, resulting in an ethically questionable level of care. Therefore, the acuity and healthcare needs of the student population must be considered when evaluating staffing needs (NASN, 2015).

School nurses straddle two statutory and regulatory systems, namely, education and health. Because school nurses practice nursing in a system focused on education, they face unique policy, funding, and supervisory issues that may present ethical dilemmas. For example, a school administrator's request of the school nurse may conflict with practice regulations, or responsibilities to the school district may restrict exemplary nursing practice. School nurses must have the skills to communicate and advocate for best practice within the healthcare and education arenas, applying appropriate ethical theories and principles to their practices.

Trends and Issues in School Nursing

School nurse service delivery is changing as technology continues to evolve. The school nurse is a member of a unique professional nursing specialty and is often the sole healthcare provider in an academic setting. Twenty-first century school nursing practice is student centered, occurring within the context of the student's family and school community (NASN, 2016c). Being aware of evolving trends in healthcare reform and practice requires school nurses to be lifelong learners.

Since the Great Recession of 2008, school districts have continued to eliminate funding for school nursing (Stanhope & Lancaster, 2014). This is concurrent with stagnation of salaries, in which the average school nurse makes more than $14,000 less than the average salary of an RN (Camera, 2016). Currently, less than half of the U.S. public schools employ a full-time school nurse and about 30% of schools have a part-time school nurse (Mangena & Maughan, 2015). Consequently, inadequate staffing due to budget cuts and stagnant funding has limited the ability to provide quality care, particularly to the most vulnerable students. The limited access to school nurses, for some students, is conflated with a lack of access to health care, which increases time out of classroom and out of school. Inevitably, these issues can have a significant impact on student academic achievement and success.

School nurses work in a complex environment filled with emerging issues and trends. Careful study will help the nurse assess the ethical and clinical issues involved as they make decisions in practice. Some current issues are as follows:

- Increase in actual incidences of violence, bullying, drug and substance abuse, teenage pregnancy

- Determining school nurse workloads and acuity of student needs

- Monitoring the integration of the Every Student Succeeds Act in advancing the role of the school nurse to support student achievement

- Using evidence-based staffing/service models to meet the needs of the school population

- Managing and assisting students with complex health needs and concerns

- Collaborating and partnering with students and the extended school community and nearby healthcare providers

- Developing new roles for school nurses within wellness/health promotion; mental/behavioral health, such as antibullying programs, online bullying, drug use and abuse, adverse childhood experiences, trauma-centered care including students impacted by violence; concussion training; care coordination; and the Affordable Care Act

- Increasing responsibility to provide health care for students who are homeless
- Increasing accountability for evidence based practice and evidence regarding impact of school health services
- Advancing education for school nurses including professional development and advanced degrees
- Collecting national data for or about school nursing practices, to promote the relevance and impact of school nursing on student health and well-being
- Eliminating pay inequities for school nurses
- Standardizing school nurse certification requirements across the United States
- Developing a school nurse education model for mentoring new practitioners
- Promoting a national platform that promotes school nurse leadership from the local to national level
- Evaluating emerging technologies, such as social media, EHRs, electronic monitoring, and telehealth, and their effects on collaboration, communication, and ethics
- Improving students and their families' access to appropriate educational health information
- Integrating complementary and alternative therapies and treatments in the school setting that are safe and appropriate, such as meditations, off-label medications, equine therapy, natural products, and so forth

Summary of the Scope of School Nursing Practice

School nurses continue to adapt their practices to an ever-changing world. Challenges continue to present themselves, as do improved tools to assist the school nurse in meeting these challenges. As technology advances, so does the school nurse's practice. More students with more complex daily health needs, as well as those requiring intermittent, on-site nursing-interventions, are in schools across America and in Department of Defense Education Activity (DoDEA) schools here and abroad. Technology is available not only as a classroom tool and for expanded school health record keeping but also to allow students with health impairments greater access to the education and socialization they are entitled to receive. The tenets of the Whole School, Whole Community, Whole Child (WSCC) model call for greater alignment, integration, and collaboration between education and health to improve each child's cognitive, physical, social, and emotional development for successful learning outcomes and wellness. The future of school nursing rests on the ability of the school nurse to successfully meet the challenges in the health and education communities.

School Nursing: Scope and Standards of Practice, 3rd Edition describes the professional responsibilities of all RNs engaged in school nursing practice, regardless of setting. As such, it can serve as a basis for a range of uses, such as

- Position recruitment announcements
- Position description creation
- New employee orientation
- Performance appraisal/evaluation
- Agency policy, protocol, and procedure development
- Competency identification and development
- Education of individuals regarding the role of school nurses
- Quality improvement systems and/or program evaluation efforts
- Development and evaluation of school nursing service delivery systems and organizational structures
- Educational offerings
- Database development, data collection, and research
- Establishing the legal standard of care
- Healthcare reimbursement and financing methodologies
- Regulatory review and revision

School nurses are uniquely positioned to enhance the quality of care and foster a national and local culture that supports the health and wellness of their school communities.

Standards of School Nursing Practice

The Standards of School Nursing Practice are authoritative statements of the duties that all school nurses are expected to perform competently. The standards published herein may be utilized as evidence of the standard of care, with the understanding that application of the standards is context dependent. The standards are subject to change with the dynamics of the nursing profession and school nursing, as new patterns of professional practice are developed and accepted by the nursing profession, the school nursing community, and the public. In addition, specific conditions and clinical circumstances may also affect the application of the standards at a given time, for example, during a natural disaster, a school lockdown or other crisis, or workload issue. The standards are subject to formal, periodic review and revision.

The competencies that accompany each standard may be evidence of compliance with the corresponding standard. The list of competencies is not exhaustive. Whether a particular standard or competency applies depends upon the circumstances. The competencies related to each of the standards identify the minimum measurable level of nursing performance of all school nurses. Experienced generalist school nurses, however, may perform competencies consistent with advanced education. Graduate-level-prepared school nurses (master's or doctoral level such as PhD, EdD, DNSc, and DNP) focus on populations, systems, complexity of issues, and growth of the specialty, so additional competencies are listed for those school nurses. In some cases, additional competencies apply both to those with graduate-level standing and to advanced practice registered nurses and are so identified. Finally, some competencies are listed just for the advanced practice registered nurse in the role of a school nurse.

Standards of Practice for School Nursing

Standard 1. Assessment

The school nurse collects pertinent data and information relative to the student and community's health or the situation.

Competencies

The school nurse:

- ► Collects pertinent data, including but not limited to demographics, social determinants of health, health disparities, and physical, functional, psychosocial, emotional, cognitive, sexual, cultural, age-related, environmental, spiritual/transpersonal, and economic assessments in a systematic, ongoing process with compassion and respect for the inherent dignity, worth, and unique attributes of every person.
- ► Recognizes the importance of the assessment parameters identified by the World Health Organization, *Healthy People 2020*, or other organizations that influence nursing practice.
- ► Integrates evidence-based knowledge from global and environmental factors into the assessment process to foster an inclusive and collaborative climate.
- ► Elicits student and community values, preferences, beliefs, expressed and unexpressed needs, and knowledge of their healthcare situation.
- ► Recognizes the impact of one's own personal attitudes, values, and beliefs on the assessment process.

- Identifies barriers to effective written, verbal, and nonverbal communication based on biological, ethnic, cultural, psychosocial, literacy, environmental, and financial considerations.
- Assesses the impact of family dynamics on the student's health and wellness.
- Engages the student and other interprofessional team members in holistic, culturally sensitive data collection.
- Prioritizes data collection based on the student's immediate condition or the anticipated needs of the student or situation.
- Uses evidence-based assessment techniques, instruments, tools, available data, information, and knowledge relevant to the situation to identify patterns and variances.
- Applies ethical, legal, privacy, and confidentiality guidelines and policies to the collection, maintenance, use, and dissemination of data and information.
- Recognizes the students and family as the authority on their own health by honoring their care preferences.
- Documents relevant data accurately and, in accordance with privacy regulations, in a manner accessible to the interprofessional team.

Additional competencies for the graduate-level-prepared school nurse

In addition to the school nurse competencies, the graduate-level-prepared school nurse:

- Assesses the effect of interactions among the student, family, community, and social systems on health and illness.
- Synthesizes the results and information leading to clinical understanding.
- Synthesizes aggregated data from multiple sources throughout the assessment process.
- Partners with populations in need, as well as with relevant health professionals, school colleagues, and other stakeholders to attach meaning to population-focused data.

Additional competencies for the advanced practice registered nurse

In addition to the competencies of the school nurse and the graduate-level-prepared school nurse, the advanced practice registered nurse:

▶ Initiates diagnostic tests and procedures relevant to the student's current status.

▶ Uses advanced assessment, knowledge, and skills to maintain, enhance, or improve health conditions.

Standard 2. Diagnosis

The school nurse analyzes assessment data to determine actual or potential diagnoses, problems, and issues.

Competencies

The school nurse:

> ▶ Identifies actual or potential risks to the health and safety of the student, family, or school community and/or barriers to their health, which may include but are not limited to interpersonal, systematic, cultural, or environmental circumstances.

> ▶ Uses assessment data, standardized classification systems, technology, and clinical decision support tools to articulate actual or potential diagnoses, problems, and issues relevant to the school populations.

> ▶ Verifies the diagnoses, problems, and issues with the individual, family, group, community, population, and interprofessional colleagues.

> ▶ Prioritizes diagnoses, problems, and issues based on mutually established goals to meet the needs of the student across the health–illness continuum.

> ▶ Documents diagnoses, problems, and issues in a manner that facilitates the determination of the expected outcomes and plan.

> ▶ Interprets the diagnoses or issues to the student, family, and appropriate school staff.

Additional competencies for the graduate-level-prepared school nurse

In addition to the competencies of the school nurse, the graduate-level-prepared school nurse:

> ▶ Uses information and communication technologies to analyze diagnostic practice patterns of nurses and other members of the interprofessional team.

> ▶ Employs aggregate-level data to articulate diagnoses, problems, and issues of students, communities, and organizational systems.

Additional competencies for the advanced practice registered nurse

In addition to the competencies of the school nurse and the graduate-level-prepared school nurse, the advanced practice registered nurse:

▶ Formulates a differential diagnosis based on assessment, history, physical examination, and diagnostic test results.

Standard 3. Outcomes Identification

The school nurse identifies expected outcomes for a plan individualized to the student or the situation.

Competencies

The school nurse:

- ▶ Engages the student, interprofessional team, and others in partnership to identify expected outcomes.
- ▶ Formulates culturally sensitive expected outcomes derived from assessments and diagnoses.
- ▶ Uses clinical expertise and current evidence-based practice to identify health risks, benefits, costs, with expected trajectory of the condition.
- ▶ Collaborates with the student and family to define expected outcomes integrating the student's culture, values, and ethical considerations.
- ▶ Generates a time frame for the attainment of expected outcomes.
- ▶ Develops expected outcomes that facilitate coordination of care.
- ▶ Modifies expected outcomes based on the evaluation of the status of the student and situation.
- ▶ Documents expected outcomes as measurable goals.
- ▶ Evaluates the actual outcomes in relation to expected outcomes, safety, and quality standards.
- ▶ Defines expected outcomes that incorporate cost and clinical effectiveness and are aligned with the outcomes identified by members of the interprofessional team.
- ▶ Differentiates outcomes that require care process interventions from those that require system-level actions.
- ▶ Integrates scientific evidence and best practices to achieve expected outcomes.
- ▶ Advocates for outcomes that reflect the student's culture, values, and ethical concerns.

Additional competencies for the graduate-level-prepared school nurse, including the APRN

In addition to the competencies of the school nurse, the graduate-level-prepared school nurse or advanced practice registered nurse:

▶ Seeks new scientific evidence and best practices to achieve expected outcomes.

▶ Synthesizes cost/benefits data and literature to promote better outcomes for school nursing activities.

▶ Acts as a resource for the school community in the development of population-based health and education outcomes.

▶ Uses trends and student outcomes to guide district planning for future school programs.

Standard 4. Planning

The school nurse develops a plan that prescribes strategies to attain expected, measurable outcomes.

Competencies

The school nurse:

▶ Develops an individualized, holistic, evidence-based plan in partnership with the student who has complex conditions and his or her interprofessional team.

▶ Establishes the plan priorities with the student and interprofessional team.

▶ Advocates for responsible and appropriate use of interventions to minimize unwarranted or unwanted treatment and/or student suffering.

▶ Prioritizes elements of the plan based on the assessment of the student's level of risk and safety needs.

▶ Applies appropriate diagnostic test findings to guide interventions relevant to student's current health status.

▶ Includes evidence-based strategies in the plan to address each of the identified diagnoses, problems, or issues. These strategies may include but are not limited to:

  ▸ Promotion and restoration of health,

  ▸ Prevention of illness, injury, and disease,

  ▸ Facilitation of healing,

  ▸ Alleviation of suffering, and

  ▸ Supportive care.

▶ Incorporates an implementation pathway that describes steps and milestones.

▶ Identifies cost and economic implications of the plan.

▶ Develops a plan that reflects compliance with current statutes, rules and regulations, and standards.

- Modifies the plan according to the ongoing assessment of the student's response and other outcome indicators.
- Documents the plan using standardized language or recognized terminology.

Additional competencies for the graduate-level-prepared school nurse

In addition to the competencies of the school nurse, the graduate-level-prepared school nurse:

- Designs strategies and tactics to meet the multifaceted and complex needs of students and the school community or others.
- Leads the design and development of interprofessional processes to address the identified diagnoses, problems, or issues.
- Designs innovative nursing practices.
- Actively participates in the development and continuous improvement of systems that support the planning process.

Additional competencies for the advanced practice registered nurse

In addition to the competencies of the school nurse and graduate-level-prepared school nurse, the advanced practice registered nurse:

- Integrates assessment strategies, diagnostic strategies, and therapeutic interventions that reflect current evidence-based knowledge and traditional, alternative, or complementary healthcare practices.

Standard 5. Implementation

The school nurse implements the identified plan.

Competencies

The school nurse:

▶ Partners with the student and family to implement the plan in a safe, effective, efficient, timely, patient-centered, and equitable manner (IOM, 2010).

▶ Integrates interprofessional collaboration in the implementation of the plan through collaboration and communication across the continuum of care.

▶ Demonstrates caring behaviors toward students to develop therapeutic relationships.

▶ Provides culturally congruent, holistic care that focuses on the student and school community and addresses and advocates for the needs of diverse populations.

▶ Uses evidence-based interventions and strategies to achieve the mutually identified goals and outcomes specific to the problem or needs.

▶ Integrates critical thinking and technology solutions to implement the nursing process to collect, measure, record, retrieve, trend, and analyze data and information to enhance nursing practice and student outcomes.

▶ Delegates according to the health, safety, and welfare of the student and considering the circumstance, person, task, direction or communication, supervision, evaluation, as well as the state nurse practice act regulations, institution, and regulatory entities while maintaining accountability for the care.

▶ Documents implementation and any modifications, including changes or omissions, of the identified plan in the appropriate health and education records.

▶ Integrates traditional, alternative and complementary healthcare practices as appropriate.

▶ Provides appropriately prescribed interventions, including medication administration and treatments, and standard of care for students in the school community.

- Responds to health issues by providing counseling and crisis intervention when required, in such areas as teen pregnancy, substance abuse, death of family members, suicide, and child neglect or abuse.
- Facilitates, with student and family input, in assessing and assuring responsible use of interventions to minimize unwarranted or unwanted treatment and student suffering.
- Facilitates utilization of systems, organizations, and community resources to lead effective change and implement the plan.
- Incorporates new knowledge and strategies to initiate changes in nursing care practices if desired outcomes are not achieved.

Additional competencies for the graduate-level-prepared school nurse

In addition to the competencies of the school nurse, the graduate-level-prepared school nurse:

- Applies quality principles, while articulating methods, tools, performance measures, and standards as they relate to implementation of the plan.
- Translates evidence into practice.
- Leads interprofessional teams to communicate, collaborate, and consult effectively.
- Demonstrates leadership skills that emphasize ethical and critical decision-making, effective working relationships, and a systems perspective.
- Serves as a consultant to provide additional insight and potential solutions to complex situations.
- Uses theory-driven approaches to effect organizational or system change.
- Participates in the development and continuous improvement of systems that support the implementation of the plan.
- Fosters organizational systems that support implementation of the plan.
- Participates in the development and implementation of written policies and procedures for the clinical services and programs addressing school health and well-being.
- Mentors other school nurses on appropriate implementation of plans.

Additional competencies for the advance practice registered nurse

In addition to the competencies of the school nurse and the graduate-level-prepared school nurse, the advanced practice registered nurse:

▶ Uses prescriptive authority, procedures, referrals, treatments, and therapies in accordance with state and federal laws and regulations.

▶ Prescribes traditional and integrative evidence-based treatments, therapies, and procedures that are compatible with the student and family's cultural preferences and norms.

▶ Prescribes evidence-based pharmacological agents and treatments according to clinical indicators and results of diagnostic and laboratory tests.

▶ Provides clinical consultation for students and professionals related to complex clinical cases to improve care and patient outcomes.

▶ Provides students and families with individually understandable information about intended effects and potential adverse effects of treatments and information about costs, alternative treatments, and procedures.

▶ Documents all prescriptive interventions, procedures, referrals, treatments, and therapies according to regulatory rules.

Standard 5A. Coordination of Care

The school nurse coordinates care delivery.

Competencies

The school nurse:

- Organizes the components of the plan.
- Collaborates with students to help manage health care based on mutually agreed-upon outcomes.
- Manages a student's care in order to reach mutually agreed-upon outcomes.
- Engages the student in self-care to achieve preferred goals for quality of life.
- Assists the student to identify alternative options for care.
- Communicates with the student, family, interprofessional team, and community-based resources to effect safe transitions in continuity of care, including the use of proper authorizations in accordance with regulations and policies.
- Advocates for the delivery of dignified culturally congruent, developmentally appropriate, and holistic care by the interprofessional team.
- Documents the coordination of care.
- Educates colleagues regarding coordination and implementation of the plan.
- Incorporates the Individualized Healthcare Plan into the student's educational day and school-sponsored activities.
- Coordinates creation and implementation of the Individualized Healthcare Plan.
- Provides leadership in the coordination of interprofessional health care for integrated delivery of school health services to achieve safe, effective, efficient, timely, patient-centered, and equitable care (IOM, 2010).

Additional competencies for the graduate-level-prepared school nurse

In addition to the competencies of the school nurse, the graduate-level-prepared school nurse:

- ▶ Manages identified student panels or populations.
- ▶ Coordinates education and healthcare systems and community resources that enhance delivery of care across continuums.
- ▶ Synthesizes data and information to support and provide necessary system and community support measures, including modifications of school environments.

Additional competencies for the advanced practice registered nurse

In addition to the competencies of the school nurse and the graduate-level-prepared school nurse, the advanced practice registered nurse:

- ▶ Serves as the student's primary care provider and coordinator of healthcare services in accordance with state and federal laws and regulations.

Standard 5B. Health Teaching and Health Promotion

The school nurse employs strategies to promote health and a safe environment.

Competencies

The school nurse:

- ▶ Provides opportunities for the student and school community to identify needed healthcare promotion, disease prevention, and self-management topics.

- ▶ Engages health promotion/health teaching in collaboration with the student's values, beliefs, health practices, developmental level, learning needs, readiness and ability to learn, language preference, spirituality, culture, and socioeconomic status.

- ▶ Uses feedback and evaluations from the student to determine the effectiveness of the employed strategies.

- ▶ Uses technologies to communicate health promotion and disease prevention information to the student and school community.

- ▶ Provides students and families with information about intended effects and potential adverse effects of the plan of care within the school setting.

- ▶ Engages consumer alliance and advocacy groups in health teaching and health promotion activities for students and the school community.

- ▶ Provides anticipatory guidance to students and families to promote health and prevent or reduce the risk of negative health outcomes.

- ▶ Promotes health, wellness, self-care, and safety through education of the school community regarding health issues.

- ▶ Collaborates with other school health professionals to provide appropriate and timely health promotion and health education to the student, family, and school community.

- ▶ Promotes health principles through the *Framework for 21st Century School Nursing Practice* and the Whole School, Whole Community, Whole Child model for students and the school community.

▶ Evaluates health information resources within the area of practice for accuracy, readability, and comprehensibility to help the school community access quality health information.

▶ Serves as a primary resource to the school community regarding health information and wellness.

▶ Conducts personalized health teaching and counseling considering comparative-effectiveness research recommendations.

▶ Participates in the evaluation of health curricula and other health instructional materials and activities.

Additional competencies for the graduate-level-prepared school nurse or the APRN

In addition to the competencies of the school nurse, the graduate-level-prepared school nurse and the advanced practice registered nurse:

▶ Designs materials and activities for school community education appropriate to age, developmental level, learning needs, readiness to learn, and cultural values and beliefs of the target audience.

▶ Synthesizes empirical evidence on risk behaviors, gender roles, learning theories, behavioral change theories, motivational theories, translational theories for evidence-based practice, epidemiology, and other related theories and frameworks when designing health education information and programs.

▶ Promotes health education and health promotion for the areas identified by the Centers for Disease Control as indications for morbidity and early mortality.

Standard 6. Evaluation

The school nurse evaluates progress toward attainment of goals and outcomes.

Competencies

The school nurse:

- ▶ Conducts a holistic, systematic, ongoing, and criterion-based evaluation of the goals and outcomes in relation to the structure, processes, and timeline prescribed in the plan.
- ▶ Collaborates with the student, family, and others involved in the care or situation in the evaluation process.
- ▶ Determines, in partnership with the student, family, and other stakeholders, the patient centeredness, effectiveness, efficiency, safety, timeliness, and equitability (IOM, 2001) of the strategies in relation to the responses to the plan and attainment of outcomes. Other defined criteria (e.g., Quality and Safety Education for Nurses) may be used as well.
- ▶ Uses ongoing assessment data to revise the diagnoses, outcomes, plan, and implementation strategies, including holistic approaches.
- ▶ Shares evaluation data and conclusions with the student, family, and other stakeholders in accordance with federal and state regulations.
- ▶ Documents the results of the evaluation.
- ▶ Participates in assessing and assuring the appropriate use of interventions to avoid or minimize unwarranted and unwanted treatment and student suffering.

Additional competencies for the graduate-level-prepared registered school nurse, including the APRN

In addition to the competencies of the school nurse, the graduate-level-prepared school nurse or advanced practice registered nurse:

- ▶ Synthesizes evaluation data from the student, family, community, population, and/or institution to determine the effectiveness of the plan.

▶ Engages in a systematic evaluation process to revise the plan to enhance its effectiveness.

▶ Uses results of the evaluation to make or recommend process, policy, procedure, or protocol revisions when warranted, especially to promote student health programs that support student learning and healthy development.

Standards of Professional Performance for School Nursing

Standard 7. Ethics
The school nurse practices ethically.

Competencies

The school nurse:

- ▶ Integrates the *Code of Ethics for Nurses with Interpretive Statements* (ANA, 2015a) and the *Code of Ethics for School Nurses* (NASN, 2016b) to guide nursing practice and articulate the moral foundation of school nursing.

- ▶ Practices with compassion and respect for the inherent autonomy, dignity, worth, and unique attributes of all people.

- ▶ Advocates for student and family rights to informed decision-making and self-determination.

- ▶ Seeks guidance in situations where the rights of the student and parent conflict with public health guidelines.

- ▶ Endorses the understanding that the primary commitment is to the student regardless of setting or situation.

- ▶ Maintains therapeutic relationships and professional boundaries.

- ▶ Advocates for the rights, health, and safety of the student and school community.

- ▶ Safeguards the privacy and confidentiality of students, their data, and information within ethical, legal, and regulatory parameters, that is, FERPA and HIPAA.

- ▶ Demonstrates professional accountability and responsibility for school nursing practice.

- Maintains competence through continued personal and professional development.

- Demonstrates commitment to self-reflection and self-care.

- Contributes to the establishment and maintenance of an ethical environment that is conducive to safe, quality health care in the educational setting.

- Advances the profession through scholarly inquiry, professional standards development, and the generation of policy.

- Collaborates with other health professionals and the public to protect human rights, promote health diplomacy, enhance cultural sensitivity and congruence, and reduce health disparities.

- Articulates nursing values to maintain personal integrity and the integrity of the profession.

- Integrates principles of social justice into school nursing practice and policy.

- Integrates caring, kindness, and respect into nursing practice.

Additional competencies for the graduate-level-prepared school nurse, including the APRN

In addition to the competencies of the school nurse, the graduate-level-prepared school nurse or the advanced practice registered nurse:

- Interprets the risks, benefits, and outcomes of policies, programs, and services for school populations and communities to administrators and others, as well as the potential impact on the delivery of health-related services.

- Advocates for the establishment and operation of an ethics committee for the school district.

- Participates in interprofessional teams that address ethical risks, benefits, and outcomes.

Standard 8. Culturally Congruent Practice

The school nurse practices in a manner that is congruent with cultural diversity and inclusion principles.

Competencies

The school nurse:

▶ Demonstrates respect, equity, and empathy in actions and interactions with all students, families, and the school community.

▶ Participates in lifelong learning to understand cultural preferences, worldview, choices, and decision-making processes of diverse school communities.

▶ Creates an inventory of one's own values, beliefs, and cultural heritage.

▶ Applies knowledge of variations in health beliefs, practices, and communication patterns in all nursing practice activities.

▶ Identifies the stage of the student's acculturation and accompanying patterns of needs and engagement.

▶ Considers the effects and impact of discrimination and oppression on practice within and among vulnerable cultural groups.

▶ Uses skills and tools that are appropriately vetted for the culture, literacy, and language of the population served.

▶ Communicates with appropriate language and behaviors, including the use of interpreters and translators in accordance with healthcare preferences.

▶ Identifies the cultural-specific meaning of interactions, terms, and content (e.g., who is the family decision-maker, appropriate terminology and salutations, communication characteristics, and appropriate written material).

▶ Respects student and family decisions based on age, tradition, belief and family influence, and stage of acculturation.

▶ Advocates for policies that promote health and prevent harm among culturally diverse, underserved, or underrepresented students and families.

- ▶ Promotes equal access to school health services, interventions, health promotion programs, enrollment in research, health, and academic education, and other opportunities.

- ▶ Educates nurse colleagues and other professionals about cultural similarities and differences of students and families in the school community.

- ▶ Promotes an ongoing safe, respectful, inclusive, culturally congruent school environment.

- ▶ Advances organizational policies, programs, services, and practice that reflect respect, equity, and values for diversity and inclusion.

- ▶ Engages students, families, key stakeholders, and others in designing and establishing internal and external cross-cultural partnerships.

- ▶ Engages in critical self-reflection to improve culturally congruent practice.

Additional competencies for the graduate-level-prepared school nurse

In addition to the competencies of the school nurse, the graduate-level-prepared school nurse:

- ▶ Evaluates tools, instruments, and services provided to culturally diverse school communities.

- ▶ Conducts research to improve health care and healthcare outcomes for culturally diverse students.

- ▶ Develops recruitment and retention strategies to achieve a multicultural workforce.

- ▶ Leads interprofessional teams to identify the cultural and language needs of students and families in the school community.

- ▶ Uses appropriate assessment tools to plan culturally appropriate interventions.

- ▶ Develops programs for school nurses and colleagues with goal of reduced disparities and improved equitable care using culturally specific interventions.

Additional competencies for the advanced practice registered nurse

In addition to the competencies of the registered nurse and graduate-level-prepared registered nurse, the advanced practice registered nurse:

▶ Promotes shared decision-making solutions in planning, prescribing, and evaluating processes when the student and family cultural preferences and norms may create incompatibility with evidence-based practice.

Standard 9. Communication

The school nurse communicates effectively in all areas of practice.

Competencies

The school nurse:

► Assesses one's own communication skills and effectiveness.

► Demonstrates cultural empathy and sensitivity when communicating.

► Assesses communication ability, health literacy, resources, and preferences of students and families to inform the interprofessional team and others.

► Uses language translation resources to ensure effective communication.

► Incorporates appropriate alternative strategies to communicate effectively with students and families who have visual, speech, language, or communication difficulties.

► Uses communication styles and methods that demonstrate caring, respect, deep listening, authenticity, and trust.

► Conveys accurate information in appropriate formats for students and families.

► Maintains communication with interprofessional team and others to facilitate safe transitions and continuity in care delivery.

► Contributes the nursing perspective in interactions with others and discussions with the interprofessional team.

► Questions care processes and decisions when they do not appear to be in the best interest of the student and family.

► Discloses concerns related to potential or actual hazards and errors in care or the practice environment to the appropriate level.

► Demonstrates continuous improvement of communication skills.

► Applies regulations pertaining to privacy and confidentiality to maintain the rights of individual students and families in all communications.

- Uses communication as a strategy to achieve nursing outcomes.
- Engages in formal and informal health counseling techniques as effective communication strategies.

Additional competencies for the graduate-level-prepared school nurse, including the APRN

In addition to the competencies of the registered nurse, the graduate-level-prepared registered nurse or advanced practice registered nurse:

- Assumes a leadership role in shaping or fashioning environments that promote healthy communication.
- Advances district wide communication systems to meet student, nursing, and administrative needs.
- Evaluates the effectiveness of district or statewide (if appropriate) communication systems.

Standard 10. Collaboration

The school nurse collaborates with key stakeholders in the conduct of nursing practice.

Competencies

The school nurse:

- ▶ Identifies the areas of expertise and contribution of other professionals and key stakeholders.
- ▶ Articulates clearly the school nurse's role and responsibilities within the team.
- ▶ Uses the unique and complementary abilities of all members of the team to optimize attainment of desired outcomes.
- ▶ Partners with the student, family, and key stakeholders to advocate for and effect change, leading to positive outcomes and quality care.
- ▶ Uses appropriate tools and techniques, including information systems and technologies, to facilitate discussion and team functions, in a manner that protects dignity, respect, privacy, and confidentiality.
- ▶ Promotes engagement through consensus building and conflict management.
- ▶ Uses effective group dynamics and strategies to enhance team performance.
- ▶ Exhibits dignity and respect when interacting with others and giving and receiving feedback.
- ▶ Partners with all stakeholders to create, implement, and evaluate a comprehensive plan.
- ▶ Adheres to standards and applicable codes of conduct that govern behavior among peers and colleagues to create a work environment that promotes cooperation, respect, and trust.
- ▶ Invites the contribution of the student, family, and key stakeholders to achieve optimal outcomes.
- ▶ Documents the outcomes and decisions of collaborative planning.

▶ Provides leadership for establishing, improving, and sustaining collaborative relationships to achieve safe, quality care for the school community.

▶ Leverages knowledge of community health systems and populations to enhance function as an effective collaborator.

Additional competencies for the graduate-level-prepared school nurse, including the APRN

In addition to the competencies of the school nurse, the graduate-level-prepared school nurse or advanced practice registered nurse:

▶ Participates in interprofessional activities, including but not limited to education, consultation, management, technological development, or research to enhance outcomes.

▶ Advances interprofessional plan-of-care documentation and communications, rationales for plan-of-care changes, and collaborative discussions to improve student outcomes.

Standard 11. Leadership

The school nurse leads within the professional practice setting and the profession.

Competencies

The school nurse:

▶ Contributes to the establishment of an environment that supports and maintains respect, trust, and dignity.

▶ Encourages innovation in practice and role performance to attain personal and professional plans, goals, and vision.

▶ Communicates to manage change and address conflict.

▶ Mentors colleagues for the advancement of school nursing practice and the nursing profession to enhance safe, quality health care.

▶ Retains accountability for delegated nursing care.

▶ Contributes to the evolution of the profession through participation in professional organizations.

▶ Influences policy to promote health for students and school communities at the local, state, and national level.

▶ Mentors colleagues in the acquisition of clinical knowledge, skills, abilities, and judgment.

▶ Engages in teamwork as a team player and team builder.

▶ Demonstrates knowledge of the roles of other school professionals and staff.

▶ Serves in key roles in the school and work settings by participating on committees, councils, and administrative teams at all levels.

▶ Inspires loyalty by valuing people as the most precious asset in an organization.

Additional competencies for the graduate-level-prepared school nurse, including the APRN

In addition to the competencies of the registered nurse, the graduate-level-prepared registered nurse or advanced practice registered nurse:

- ▶ Influences decision-making bodies to improve the professional practice environment and student, family, and school community outcomes.

- ▶ Provides direction to enhance the effectiveness of the interprofessional team.

- ▶ Promotes advanced practice nursing and role development by interpreting its role for students, families, the school community, and policy makers.

- ▶ Models expert practice to interprofessional team members and the school community.

- ▶ Establishes protocols or guidelines to reflect evidence-based practice, to reflect accepted changes in care management, or to address emerging problems.

Standard 12. Education

The school nurse seeks knowledge and competence that reflects current nursing practice and promotes futuristic thinking.

Competencies

The school nurse:

- ▶ Identifies learning needs based on nursing knowledge, the various roles the nurse may assume, and the changing needs of the population within the school setting.

- ▶ Participates in ongoing educational activities related to school nursing and interprofessional knowledge bases and professional topics.

- ▶ Mentors nurses new to the school nursing role for the purpose of ensuring successful enculturation, orientation, induction, and emotional support.

- ▶ Demonstrates a commitment to lifelong learning through self-reflection and inquiry for learning and personal growth.

- ▶ Seeks experiences that reflect current practice to maintain and advance knowledge, skills, abilities, attitudes, and judgment in clinical practice or role performance.

- ▶ Acquires knowledge, skills, and abilities relative to the school nurse role, the population of students, their families, and the school community, as well as the global or local health situation.

- ▶ Participates in formal consultations or informal discussions to address issues in nursing practice and school nursing practice as an application of education and knowledge.

- ▶ Identifies modifications or accommodations needed in the delivery of education, based on student and family members' needs.

- ▶ Shares educational findings, experiences, and ideas with health and education colleagues.

- ▶ Supports acculturation of school nurses new to their roles by role modeling, encouraging, and sharing pertinent information relative to optimal care delivery.

- ▶ Encourages the sharing of pertinent information relative to optimal healthcare delivery in an educational setting.

- ▶ Facilitates a work environment supportive of ongoing education of nursing and healthcare professionals.

- ▶ Maintains a professional portfolio that provides evidence of individual competence and lifelong learning.

- ▶ Promotes communication of information and advancement of the profession through writing, publishing, and presentations for professional or lay audiences.

- ▶ Maintains national certification and state credentialing when applicable.

Additional competencies for the graduate-level-prepared school nurse, including the APRN

In addition to the competencies of the school nurse, the graduate-level-prepared school nurse or the advanced practice registered nurse:

- ▶ Uses current healthcare research findings and other evidence to expand clinical knowledge, skills, abilities, and judgments for the enhancement of role performance and to increase knowledge of professional issues.

- ▶ Uses current needs and healthcare research to plan, develop, design, implement, and evaluate professional development or higher education programs at the local, state, and national levels.

- ▶ Provides educational opportunities for colleagues and others.

Standard 13. Evidence-Based Practice and Research

The school nurse integrates evidence and research findings into practice.

Competencies

The school nurse:

▶ Articulates the values of research and its application relative to the healthcare setting and practice of school nursing.

▶ Identifies questions in the healthcare setting and school nurse practice that may be resolved by nursing research.

▶ Uses current evidence-based knowledge, including research findings, to promote further research and guide practice.

▶ Incorporates evidence-based recommendations when initiating changes in school nursing practice.

▶ Participates in the formulation of evidence-based practice through research.

▶ Promotes ethical principles of research in all nursing practice, with particular attention to school nursing and its healthcare setting.

▶ Appraises nursing research for optimal application in school nurse practice and the healthcare setting.

▶ Shares peer-reviewed research findings with colleagues to integrate knowledge into school nursing practice.

▶ Collaborates with researchers from outside the educational system.

▶ Participates in data collection such as surveys, pilot projects, and formal studies.

▶ Engages in basic analysis and interpretation of research for application to practice.

▶ Complies with institutional, district, state, and federal policies regarding the safe conduct of research.

Additional competencies for the graduate-level-prepared school nurse, including the APRN

In addition to the competencies of the school nurse, the graduate-level-prepared school nurse or advanced practice registered nurse:

▶ Integrates current, research-based practice in all settings.

▶ Uses current healthcare research findings and other evidence to expand knowledge, skills, abilities, and judgment; to enhance role performance; and to increase knowledge of professional issues.

▶ Uses critical thinking skills to connect theory and research to school nurse practice.

▶ Integrates nursing research to improve quality in school nursing practice.

▶ Contributes to nursing knowledge by conducting or synthesizing research and other evidence that discovers, examines, and evaluates current practice, knowledge, theories, criteria, and creative approaches to improve healthcare outcomes, with special emphasis on school nursing.

▶ Encourages other nurses to develop research skills by participating in school health research activities on a local, state, national, and global scale.

▶ Performs rigorous critique of evidence derived from databases to generate meaningful evidence for school nursing practice.

▶ Advocates for the ethical conduct of research and translational scholarship with particular attention to the protection of the student as a research participant.

▶ Promotes a climate of collaborative research and clinical inquiry.

▶ Disseminates evidence-based practice outcomes and research findings through activities such as presentations, publications, consultation, and journal clubs.

Standard 14. Quality of Practice

The school nurse contributes to quality nursing practice.

Competencies

The school nurse:

▶ Ensures that nursing practice is safe, effective, efficient, equitable, timely, and patient centered (IOM, 1999, 2001).

▶ Identifies barriers and opportunities to improve healthcare safety, effectiveness, efficiency, equitability, timeliness, and student centeredness.

▶ Recommends strategies to improve school nursing quality.

▶ Uses creativity and innovation to enhance school nursing care.

▶ Participates in quality improvement initiatives.

▶ Collects data to monitor the quality of school nursing practice.

▶ Contributes in efforts to improve healthcare efficiency.

▶ Provides critical review and/or evaluation of policies, procedures, and guidelines to improve the quality of health care and delivery of school health services.

▶ Engages in formal and informal peer review processes.

▶ Collaborates with the interprofessional team to implement quality improvement plans and interventions.

▶ Documents school nursing practice in a manner that supports quality and performance improvement initiatives.

▶ Achieves professional certification, such as becoming a National Certified School Nurse.

▶ Incorporates evidence into school nursing practice to improve outcomes.

Additional competencies for the graduate-level-prepared school nurse

In addition to the competencies for the school nurse, the graduate-level-prepared school nurse:

- ► Analyzes trends in healthcare quality data, including examination of cultural influences and factors.
- ► Designs innovations to improve health and education outcomes.
- ► Provides leadership in the design and implementation of quality improvement initiatives.
- ► Promotes a practice environment that supports evidence-based health care and school health services delivery.
- ► Contributes to school nursing and interprofessional knowledge through scientific inquiry.
- ► Encourages professional or advanced specialty certification.
- ► Engages in development, implementation, evaluation, and/or revision of policies, procedures, and guidelines to improve healthcare quality.
- ► Uses data and information in system-level decision-making.
- ► Influences the organizational system to improve outcomes.
- ► Designs quality improvement studies, research, initiatives, and programs to improve health outcomes in diverse school community settings.
- ► Uses available benchmarks as a means to evaluate practice at the individual, departmental, or organizational level.

Additional competencies for the advanced practice registered nurse

In addition to the competencies for the school nurse and graduate-level-prepared school nurse, the advanced practice registered nurse:

▶ Engages in comparison evaluations of the effectiveness and efficacy of diagnostic tests, clinical procedures and therapies, and treatment plans, in partnership with students and families, to optimize health and healthcare quality.

▶ Applies knowledge obtained from advanced preparation, as well as current research and evidence-based information, to clinical decision-making at the point of care to achieve optimal health outcomes.

Standard 15. Professional Practice Evaluation

The school nurse evaluates one's own and others' nursing practice.

Competencies

The school nurse:

- ▶ Engages in self-reflection and self-evaluation of nursing practice on a regular basis, identifying areas of strength as well as areas in which professional growth would be beneficial.

- ▶ Adheres to the guidance about professional practice as specified in *School Nursing: Scope and Standards of Practice, Code of Ethics for Nurses with Interpretive Statements*, and *NASN Code of Ethics for School Nurses*.

- ▶ Ensures that nursing practice is consistent with regulatory requirements pertaining to licensure, relevant statutes, rules, and regulations.

- ▶ Uses organizational policies and procedures to guide professional practice, including use of accepted tools in self-evaluation and peer evaluation.

- ▶ Influences organizational policies and procedures to promote inter-professional evidence-based practice.

- ▶ Provides evidence for practice decisions and actions as part of the formal and informal evaluation processes.

- ▶ Seeks formal and informal feedback regarding one's own practice from students and families, peers, colleagues, supervisors, and others.

- ▶ Provides peers and others with formal and informal constructive feedback regarding their practice or role performance.

- ▶ Takes action to achieve goals identified during the evaluation process.

Standard 16. Resource Utilization

The school nurse utilizes appropriate resources to plan, provide, and sustain evidence-based nursing services that are safe, effective, and fiscally responsible.

Competencies

The school nurse:

▶ Assesses student care needs and resources available to achieve desired outcomes.

▶ Assists in factoring costs, risks, and benefits in decisions about care and delivery of school health services, including health promotion, health education, and maintaining a healthy and safe environment.

▶ Assists the student and family in identifying and securing appropriate services to address needs across the healthcare continuum.

▶ Delegates in accordance with applicable legal and policy parameters, such as the nurse practice acts, NASN *Principles of Practice* and the NCSBN *National Guidelines for Nursing Delegation.*

▶ Identifies the impact of resource allocation on the potential for harm, complexity of the task, and desired outcomes.

▶ Advocates for resources that support and enhance school nursing practice and delivery of school health services.

▶ Integrates appropriate and available telehealth and mobile health technologies into practice to promote positive interactions between students and their families and care providers.

▶ Uses organizational and community resources to implement interprofessional plans.

▶ Addresses discriminatory healthcare practices and the impact on resource allocation.

▶ Documents all aspects of resource utilization, including delegation and staff training.

Additional competencies for the graduate-level-prepared school nurse, including the APRN

In addition to the competencies of the registered nurse, the graduate-level-prepared registered nurse and advanced practice registered nurse:

▶ Designs innovative solutions to use resources effectively and maintain quality.

▶ Provides evaluation strategies that address cost effectiveness, cost–benefit, and efficiency factors associated with school nursing practice.

▶ Assumes complex and advanced leadership roles to initiate and guide change.

▶ Engages organizational and community resources to formulate and implement interprofessional collaborative plans.

Standard 17. Environmental Health

The school nurse practices in an environmentally safe and healthy manner.

Competencies

The school nurse:

- ▶ Promotes a safe and healthy workplace and professional practice environment.
- ▶ Uses environmental health concepts in practice.
- ▶ Assesses the environment to identify risk factors including safe school nursing staff levels, food security, sound, odor, chemicals, mold, noise, and light.
- ▶ Reduces environmental health risks to self, colleagues, and students.
- ▶ Communicates information about environmental health risks and exposure reduction strategies.
- ▶ Advocates for the safe, judicious, and appropriate use and disposal of products in health care.
- ▶ Incorporates technologies to promote safe practice environments.
- ▶ Uses products or treatments consistent with evidence-based practice to reduce environmental threats.
- ▶ Participates in developing strategies to promote healthy communities and practice environments.
- ▶ Maintains current knowledge of environmental health concepts, such as implementation of environmental health strategies.
- ▶ Creates partnerships promoting sustainable environmental health policies, including efforts to promote access.

Additional competencies for the graduate-level-prepared school nurse, including the APRN

In addition to the competencies of the registered nurse, the graduate-level-prepared registered nurse or advanced practice registered nurse:

▶ Analyzes the impact of social, political, and economic influences on the global environment and human health experience in schools for strategic planning.

▶ Leads school nurses in advocating for and implementing environmental health principles in school nursing practice.

▶ Creates partnerships that promote sustainable global environmental health policies and conditions that focus on prevention of hazards to people and the natural environment (ANA, 2007).

Standard 18. Program Management

The school nurse directs the health services program within the school and community that includes evidence-based practice and accountability measures for quality, student health, and learning outcomes.

Competencies

The school nurse:

- ▶ Identifies educational requirements and needed supports for each member of the school healthcare team (e.g., health aide, licensed practice nurse, licensed vocational nurse, or other nurses).

- ▶ Establishes the system of communication and access to communication for the healthcare team members within the school community.

- ▶ Designs a process for team members to have continuous access to evidence-based practices and guidelines.

- ▶ Determines how the school healthcare team will develop, implement, monitor, and evaluate a shared plan of care that is family centered.

- ▶ Develops interagency partnerships that support student health and education goals.

- ▶ Promotes stakeholder participation for system of care analysis of student outcomes and continuing performance improvement.

- ▶ Advocates for the needs of individual students and the school community.

- ▶ Conducts health needs assessments of the school environment to identify current health problems and identify the need for health services programming.

- ▶ Implements needed health programs using a program planning process.

- ▶ Communicates student and school community outcomes and the school health program to the community, administrators, and the school board and key stakeholders.

- ▶ Supervises the healthcare team members, including unlicensed assistive personnel (UAPs), as appropriate following legal requirements in the school setting, to include orientation, training, and documentation of competency.

▶ Interprets the role of the school nurse and school health service program needs to the school and community.

▶ Coordinates creation and implementation of the emergency action and disaster preparedness plans.

▶ Serves on school and district health and wellness committees.

▶ Acts as a resource for coordinated school health programs as described by the Whole School, Whole Community, Whole Child Model (ASCD & CDC, 2014).

▶ Adopts available technology appropriate to the work setting.

▶ Leverages cooperation among families, schools, and communities on public health issues.

▶ Acquires knowledge through participation in formal or informal consultation to address issues in school nursing practice.

Additional competencies for the graduate-level-prepared school nurse, including the APRN

In addition to the competencies of the registered nurse, the graduate-level-prepared registered nurse or advanced practice registered nurse:

▶ Serves as a mentor and resource to others on effective program management.

▶ Synthesizes clinical data, theoretical frameworks, and evidence when providing consultation.

▶ Initiates changes throughout the healthcare delivery system, as appropriate, using the results of school health environmental needs assessments, analysis of evaluation data, and quality-of-care activities.

▶ Develops health policies and procedures in collaboration with school administrators, local school boards, and local departments of health.

▶ Coordinates implementation of health policies and procedures in collaboration with district administrators, local school boards, and board of education.

▶ Identifies appropriate funding sources for school district nursing and health services.

▶ Develops school health services budget including provisions for staffing, equipment, and resources.

▶ Demonstrates knowledge of existing school health programs and current health trends that may affect health care; the sources of funds for such programs; and local, state, and federal laws governing each.

▶ Supervises school nurses and the healthcare team across the district, where applicable.

▶ Leads public health efforts across the school community.

▶ Implements effective strategies in collaboration with professional nursing organizations to exert influence with the legislative process at state and national levels related to student health issues and trends.

▶ Uses the national dataset developed by the professional organization to monitor school health services and concerns in collaboration with public health partners, the population, the interdisciplinary team, and other stakeholders.

Glossary

Ability. A characteristic of nursing competency that describes the capacity to act effectively. It requires listening, integrity, knowledge of one's strengths and weaknesses, positive self-regard, emotional intelligence, and openness to feedback.

Acculturation. The acquisition of a first culture that is essential to survival.

Advanced practice registered nurse (APRN). A nurse who has completed an accredited graduate-level education that prepares her or him for the role of certified nurse practitioner, certified registered nurse anesthetist, certified midwife, or clinical nurse specialist; has passed a national certification examination that measures the APRN role and population-focused competencies; maintains continued competence as evidenced by recertification; and is licensed to practice as an APRN.

Aggregate. A group of students or persons in the school with a similar trait, for example, grade, race, and gender.

Assessment. The first step of the nursing process in which data about the student is systematically and comprehensively collected and analyzed to formulate a nursing diagnosis or diagnoses.

Autonomy. The capacity of a nurse to determine own actions through independent choice, including demonstration of competence within the full scope of nursing practice.

Coaching. Use of skills similar to mentoring but is more limited and aims to provide a new school nurse with skills to meet tasks and challenges; seeks to encourage own approach and promotes best practices.

Code of Ethics (nursing). A list of provisions that makes explicit the primary goals, values, and obligations of the nursing profession and expresses its values, duties, and commitments to the society of which it is a part. In the United

States, nurses abide by and adhere to *Code of Ethics for Nurses with Interpretive Statements* (ANA, 2015).

Collaboration. A professional healthcare partnership grounded in a reciprocal and respectful recognition and acceptance of each partner's unique expertise, power, and sphere of influence and responsibilities; the commonality of goals; the mutual safeguarding of the legitimate interest of each party; and the advantages of such a relationship.

Competency. An expected and measurable level of nursing performance that integrates knowledge, skills, abilities, and judgment, based on established scientific knowledge and expectations for nursing practice. Competency statements are specific, measurable elements that interpret, explain, and facilitate practical use of the standard.

Complexity. An attribute that represents multifactorial influence on a problem or solution; it represents simultaneously occurring problems and issues requiring appropriate intervention.

Crisis management plan. Plan developed by multiple constituencies in preparation for a school-wide or community disaster or crisis.

Culture of health. A way of thinking, behaving, or working that puts well-being at the center of every life.

Delegation. The assignment of the performance of a nursing activity to a nonnurse. The school nurse, who, after assessment of the individual's capabilities, makes a prudent decision regarding the advisability of delegation. Accountability remains with the registered nurse; state laws and regulations and school regulations must be followed; and standards of school nursing practice must be upheld. The registered nurse may decide against delegation for safety, regulatory, and legal issues; school staffing or student health status issues; or unlicensed assistive personnel (UAP) competence or ability.

Diagnosis. The second step of the nursing process in which the analysis of assessed data results in a clinical judgment expressed as a statement of the student's response to actual or potential health needs or conditions. The diagnosis provides the basis for determining a plan to achieve expected outcomes.

Emergency Care (or Action) Plan (ECP or EAP). A child-specific guide for school staff to facilitate quick and appropriate response for an individual student emergency.

Enculturation. The merging of a first culture with two or more cultures (i.e., nursing with school nursing).

Evaluation. The sixth and final step of the nursing process in which the nurse systematically and continuously appraises progress toward attainment of outcomes; measurable elements that interpret, explain, and facilitate practical use of the standard.

Evidence-based practice. A problem-solving approach to health care using healthcare provider expertise, the best scientific evidence, and the consumer's values and preference to determine and guide the plan of care.

Expected outcomes. End results that are measurable, desirable, and observable and translate into observable behaviors.

Family. The family of origin or significant others as identified by the student.

Formal learning. A means of integrating knowledge, skills, abilities, and judgment, which most often occurs in structured, academic, and professional development environments.

Graduate-level-prepared school nurse. A nursing leader in school nursing and health, prepared at the master's or doctoral level, who possesses specialized knowledge and skills in school nursing, public health, organization and management, health education, health promotion, administration, or other areas of study necessary to promote the health and academic success of the student and professional school nursing practice.

Health. An experience that is often expressed in terms of wellness and illness and may occur in the presence or absence of disease or injury.

Health care. The prevention, treatment, and management of illness; the preservation of mental and physical well-being; and the promotion of health through services offered by a healthcare provider or health professional.

Healthcare consumer. The student, family, group, school community, or population who is the focus of attention and to whom the school nurse is providing services as sanctioned by state regulatory bodies. In school nursing, the student and those who influence students such as the family, school community, the larger surrounding community, aggregates within the school population, or the entire school population are the healthcare consumers.

Healthcare provider. A person with special education and expertise who provides healthcare services or assistance to students and their families.

Healthy work environment. An employment atmosphere characterized by optimal physical, psychological, economic, and political conditions conducive to optimal productivity, including worker and the school community's safety, employer support and encouragement, absence of undue stress, and reasonable and sustainable staffing conditions and caseloads.

Holistic care. Integration of body–mind–spirit–sexual–cultural–social–energetic–environmental principles to promote health and well-being and actualize human potential.

Implementation. The fifth step of the nursing process in which the nurse acts to bring about the plan. In the standards of practice, the process of implementation has several components that include coordination of care; health teaching and health promotion; consultation; and, for the APRN, prescriptive authority and treatment, when allowed.

Individual Family Service Plan (IFSP). A multidisciplinary plan, specific to infants, toddlers, and preschoolers with special needs, and inclusive of their families.

Individualized Educational (Program) Plan (IEPP/IEP). A multidisciplinary and multifaceted plan for students 5 through 21 years (older in some states) who meet special education program requirements under state and federal law.

Individualized Healthcare Plan (IHP). A plan of care written by the registered nurse for a student with or at risk for physical or mental health needs.

Informal learning. A means of integrating knowledge, skills, abilities, and judgment into experiential insights gained in work, community, home, and other settings.

Interprofessional. Reliant on the overlapping knowledge, skills, and abilities of each professional team member. This can drive synergistic effects by which outcomes are enhanced and become more comprehensive than a simple aggregation of the individual efforts of the team members.

Interprofessional collaboration. Working together with others as appropriate to improve health and academic outcomes.

Judgment. A characteristic of nursing competency that includes critical thinking, problem solving, ethical reasoning, and decision-making.

Knowledge. A characteristic of nursing competency that encompasses thinking, understanding of science and humanities, professional standards of practice, and insights gained from practical experiences, personal capabilities, and leadership performance.

Liaison. A person whose function it is to maintain communication between or among individuals and an organization, parts of an organization, or between two or more organizations acting together for a common purpose.

Mentoring. Power-free, often long-term, relationship using skills similar to coaching with the goal of professional development. Advice may be more directive and always confidential.

Multidisciplinary team. A team of school or community professionals with a variety of skills, abilities, and disciplinary backgrounds who work together for a common purpose. In the context of the school, this goal is to achieve the best academic and/or health outcomes for students, their families, or others within the school community.

National Association of School Nurses (NASN). A professional organization serving the needs of school nurses nationally and internationally. As such, the NASN supports the health and educational success of children and youth by developing and providing leadership to advance school nursing practice by specialized registered nurses. As the expert voice for school nurses, the organization has the following as its core values: scholarship, excellence, collegiality, and diversity.

Nursing. The protection, promotion, and optimization of health and abilities, prevention of illness and injury, facilitation of healing, alleviation of suffering through the diagnosis and treatment of human response, and advocacy in the care of individuals, families, groups, communities, and populations.

Nursing process. A circular, continuous, and dynamic critical-thinking process comprised of six steps that is client centered, interpersonal, collaborative, and universally applicable. The six steps are assessment, diagnosis, outcomes identification, planning, implementation, and evaluation. The nursing process encompasses all significant actions taken by registered nurses and forms the foundation of the school nurse's decision-making.

Outcomes identification. The third step of the nursing process wherein measurable, expected, realistic, and attainable expectations for the student are stipulated.

Peer review. Collegial process for accountability in practice that included both interprofessional and intraprofessional collaboration.

Planning. The fourth step of the nursing process in which the nurse formulates a comprehensive outline of care to be implemented for attainment of specific measurable outcomes. In school nursing, examples are the Individualized

Healthcare Plan (IHP), the Americans with Disabilities Act (504 Plan), the Individualized Educational Program Plan (IEPP) from the Individuals with Disabilities in Education Act, the Emergency Care Plan (ECP), and others.

Population. A group of persons who have identified similarities and includes aggregates and communities.

Registered nurse (RN). An individual registered or licensed by a state, commonwealth, territory, government, or other regulatory body to practice as a registered nurse.

School. An institution, organization, or group dedicated to the provision of educational services for children and youth from birth through age 21 or older. Schools include public, private, and military entities.

School community. All those who study, work in, or are formally affiliated with a school district or school setting. The school community is expanded, when appropriate, to community agencies, faith-based groups, students' families, and others.

School nurse administrator. A professional registered school nurse who also is recognized or employed in the capacity of supervision of school nurses or others and expected to carry out school health or other administrative responsibilities in the school setting, such as coordination of school health services across the school district, development of school health policies and procedures, establishment of professional development for school nurses, development of school health budgets, and evaluation of school health programs.

School nursing. School nursing, a specialized practice of nursing, protects and promotes student health, facilitates optimal development, and advances academic success. School nurses, grounded in ethical and evidence-based practice, are the leaders who bridge health care and education, provide care coordination, advocate for quality student-centered care, and collaborate to design systems that allow individuals and communities to develop their full potentials (NASN, 2017).

Scope of school nursing practice. A statement describing the complex and unique practice of the school nurse, including its considerable depth and breadth. The scope statement describes the "who," "what," "where," "when," "why," and "how" of school nursing practice. The statement is intended for those who practice school nursing in the United States and its territories and in Department of Defense Education Activity (DoDEA) locations around the world and for all constituencies.

Section 504 Accommodation Plan. An interprofessional plan developed in accordance with Section 504 of the Rehabilitative Act of 1973 to assure that physical and mental health along with other educational accommodations, are implemented for children with disabilities.

Skills. A characteristic of nursing competency that includes psychomotor, communication, interpersonal, and diagnostic skills.

Social determinants of health. The influence on outcomes by a person's social environment, including educational level, neighborhood, socioeconomic status and social supports, and access to health care.

Stakeholders. Person(s) with an interest or concern related to school health, health services, or school nursing.

Standards. Authoritative statements of the duties that all registered nurses, regardless of role, population, or specialty, are expected to perform. Within school nursing, standards are the professional expectations that guide the practice of school nursing.

Student. The healthcare consumer for a school nurse; a youth attending pre-kindergarten through Grade 12 or up to 21 years of age if identified as a student with special needs under the Individuals with Disabilities Education Act.

System. Any group of interacting, interrelated, or interdependent elements forming a complex whole.

Transition plan. A multidisciplinary plan designed to facilitate smooth transition among and between schools or school levels for students with special needs.

Unlicensed assistive personnel (UAP). A person without a nursing license who has been delegated certain appropriate, routine, standardized nursing tasks by a registered nurse.

Wellness. Integrated, congruent functioning aimed toward reaching one's highest potential (ANA & AHNA, 2013).

References and Bibliography

American Academy of Pediatrics, Council of School Health. (2016). The role of the school nurse in providing school health services. *Pediatrics 137*(6). doi: 10.1542/peds.2016-0852. Retrieved from http://pediatrics.aappublications.org/content/early/2016/05/19/peds .2016-0852.

American Nurses Association (ANA). (1983). *Standards of school nursing practice.* Kansas City, MO: Author.

American Nurses Association (ANA). (2010). *Nursing's social policy statement.* Silver Spring, MD: Nursebooks.org.

American Nurses Association (ANA). (2013). *Public health nursing: Scope and standards of practice.* Silver Spring, MD: Nursebooks.org.

American Nurses Association (ANA). (2015a). *Code of ethics for nurses with interpretive statements.* Silver Spring, MD: Nursebooks.org.

American Nurses Association (ANA). (2015b). *Nursing: Scope and standards of practice* (3rd ed.). Silver Spring, MD: Nursebooks.org.

American Nurses Association (ANA). (2016). *Nursing administration: Scope and standards of practice.* Silver Spring, MD: Nursebooks.org.

American Nurses Association (ANA) & American Holistic Nursing Association (AHNA). (2013). *Holistic nursing: Scope and standards of practice.* Silver Springs, MD: Nursebooks.org.

APRN Joint Dialog Group. (2008). *Consensus model for APRN regulation: Licensure, accreditation, certification, and education.* Retrieved from http://www.nursingworld.org/DocumentVault /APRN-Resource-Section/ConsensusModelforAPRNRegulation.aspx.

ASCD & U.S. *Centers for Disease Control and Prevention* (CDC). (2014). *Whole School, Whole Community, Whole Child: A collaborative approach to learning and health.* Alexandria, VA: ASCD and CDC. Retrieved from http://www.ascd.org/ASCD/pdf/siteASCD/publications /wholechild/wscc-a-collaborative-approach.pdf.

Barden, C., Cassidy, S., & Cardin, S. (Eds.). (2016). *AACN standards for establishing and sustaining healthy work environments: A journey to excellence* (2nd ed.). Aliso Veijo, CA: AACN. Retrieved from http://www.aacn.org/wd/hwe/docs/hwestandards.pdf.

Bultas, M. W., & McLaughlin, L. (2013). Using evidence-based practice in the school health room. *NASN School Nurse, 28,* 34–40.

Camera, L. (2016, March 23). Many school districts do not have enough school nurses. *US News and World Report.* Retrieved from http://www.usnews.com/news/articles/2016-03-23 /the-school-nurse-scourge.

Carr, B., & Knutson, S. (2015). Culturally competent school nursing practice. *NASN School Nurse, 30,* 336–342.

Castronovo, M. A., Pullizzi, A., & Evans, S. (2016). Nurse bullying: A review and proposed solution. *Nursing Outlook, 64,* 208–214.

Centers for Disease Control and Prevention. (CDC). (2015). *Components of the Whole School, Whole Community, Whole Child.* Retrieved from http:www.cdc.gov/healthyschools/wscc/components.thm.

Chinn, P., & Kramer, M. K. (2008). *Integrated theory and knowledge development in nursing* (7th ed.). St. Louis, MO: Mosby.

Cowell, J. M. (2016a). Population health: Considerations for school health research and practice. *The Journal of School Nursing, 32,* 226–228.

Cowell, J. M. (2016b). What makes nursing work, *The Journal of School Nursing, 32,* 6–7.

Cowell, J. M., & Bergren, M. D. (2016). Are school nurses victims of bullying? *The Journal of School Nursing, 32,* 302–303.

Dolansky, M. A., & Moore, S. M. (2013). Quality and Safety Education for Nurses (QSEN): The key is systems thinking. *Online Journal of Issues in Nursing, 18,* 1–12.

Erwin, K., Clark, S., & Mercer, S. E. (2014). Providing health services for children with special health needs on out-of-state field trips. *Journal of School Nursing, 29,* 84–88.

Fowler, M. D. (2015). *Guide to the code of ethics for nurses: Interpretation and application.* Silver Spring, MD: Nursebooks.org.

Galemore, C. A., & Sheetz, A. H. (2015). IEP, IHP, and Section 504 primer for new school nurses. *NASN School Nurse, 30,* 85–88.

Haffke, L. M., Damm, P., & Cross, B. (2014). School nurses race to the top: The pilot year of how one district's school nurses revised their evaluation process. *The Journal of School Nursing, 30,* 404–410.

Institute of Medicine. (1999). *To err is human: Building a safer health system.* Washington, DC: The National Academies Press.

Institute of Medicine. (2001). *Crossing the quality chasm: A new health system for the 21st century.* Committee on Quality Health Care in America. Washington, DC: The National Academies Press.

Institute of Medicine. (2003). *Health professions education: A bridge to quality.* Washington, DC: The National Academies Press.

Institute of Medicine. (2010). *The future of nursing: Leading change, advancing health.* Washington, DC: National Academies Press.

Joint Committee of the National Education Association and the American Medical Association. (1941). *The nurse in the school.* Washington, DC: National Education Association and American Medical Association.

Kendall-Gallagher, D., Aiken, L. H., Sloane, D. M., & Cimotti, J. P. (2011). Nurse specialty certification, inpatient mortality, and failure to rescue. *Journal of Nursing Scholarship, 43,* 188–194.

Lewellen, T. C., Hunt, H., Potts-Datema, W., Zaza, S., & Giles, W. (2015). The Whole School, Whole Community, Whole Child model: A new approach for improving educational attainment and healthy development for students. *Journal of School Health, 85,* 729–739.

Luthy, K. E., Houle, K., Beckstrand, R. L., Macintosh, J., & Lakin, R. G. (2013). Vaccination perceptions and barriers of school employees: A pilot study. *The Journal of School Nursing, 29,* 284–293.

Mangena, A. S., & Maughan, E. (2015). The 2015 NASN school nurse survey. *NASN School Nurse, November,* 329–335.

Marion, L., Douglas, M., Lavin, M. A., Barr, N., Gazaway, S., Thomas, E., & Bickford, C. (2016). Implementing the new ANA standard 8: Culturally congruent practice. *OJIN: The Online Journal of Issues in Nursing, 21*.

Mason, D., Jones, D., Roy, C., & Sullivan, C. (2015). Commonalities of nurse-designed models of health care. *Nursing Outlook, 63*, 540–553.

Mazer, M. E., Jacobson Vann, J. C., Lamanna, B. F., & Davison, J. (2014). Reducing children's exposure to school bus diesel exhaust in one school district in North Carolina. *The Journal of School Nursing, 30*, 88–96.

McClanahan, R., & Weismuller, P. C. (2015). School nurses and care coordination for children with complex needs: An integrative review. *The Journal of School Nursing, 31*, 34–43.

McDaniel, K. H., Overman, M., Guttu, M., & Engelke, M. K. (2013). School nurse evaluations: Making the process meaningful and motivational. *The Journal of School Nursing, 29*, 19–30.

National Association of School Nurses (NASN). (2014a). Nursing delegation in the school setting [Position statement]. Retrieved from http://www.nasn.org/ToolsResources/Delegation.

National Association of School Nurses. (2014b). Environmental health in the school setting: The role of the school nurse. Retrieved from http://www.nasn,org/ToolsResources/Environmentalhealth.

National Association of School Nurses (NASN). (2016a). Education, licensure and certification of school nurses [Position statement]. Retrieved from http://www.nasn.org/PolicyAdvocacy/PositionDocuments/NASNPositionStatements/tabid/237/smid/824/ArticleId/26/Default.aspx.

National Association of School Nurses (NASN). (2016b). Code of ethics for school nurses. Retrieved from https://www.nasn.org/RoleCareer/CodeofEthics.

National Association of School Nurses. (2016c). *Framework for 21st Century School Nursing Practice*: National Association of School Nurses. *NASN School Nurse, 31*, 45–53.

National Association of School Nurses (NASN). (2016d). School nursing and school based health centers: Working together for student success [Fact sheet]. http://www.nasn.org/portals/0/advocacy/School_Nursing_and_School-Based_Health_Centers.pdf.

National Association of School Nurses (NASN). (2016e). The Role of the 21st Century School Nurse. Retrieved from https://schoolnursenet.nasn.org/blogs/nasn-profile/2017/03/13/the-role-of-the-21st-century-school-nurse.

National Education Association (NEA), Department of School Nurses. (1970). *Standards for school nurse services*. Washington, DC: Author.

Nightingale, F. (1860/1969). *Notes on nursing: What it is and what it is not*. New York, NY: Dover Publications.

Olsen, H. M., Hudson, S. D., & Thompson, D. (2008). Developing a playground injury prevention plan. *The Journal of School Nursing, 27*, 131–137.

Proctor, S. (2013). Standards of practice: What they are and how to use them. In Selekman, J. (Ed.), *School nursing: A comprehensive text* (2nd ed., pp. 48–78). Philadelphia: F.A. Davis.

Radis, M. E., Updegrove, S. C., Somsel, A., & Crowley, A. A. (2015). Negotiating access to health information to promote students' health. *The Journal of School Nursing, 32*, 81–85.

Rains, C. S., & Robinson, B. (2012). School nurses and athletic trainers team up on emergency planning. *The Journal of School Nursing, 27*, 136–142.

Rosenblum, R. K., & Sprague-McRae, J. (2014). Using principles of quality and safety education for nurses in school nurse continuing education. *Journal of School Nursing, 30*, 97–102.

Sampson, C. H., & Galemore, C. A. (2012). What every school nurse needs to know about Section 504 eligibility. *NASN School Nurse, 27*, 88–93.

Stanhope, M., & Lancester, J. (2014). *Foundations of nursing in the community: Community oriented practice.* St. Louis, Missouri: Elsevier/Mosby.

Wold, S. J., & Selekman, J. (2013). Frameworks and models for school nursing practice. In Selekman, J. (Ed.), *School nursing: A Comprehensive Text* (2nd ed., pp. 79–108). Philadelphia, PA: F.A. Davis.

Wolfe, L. C. (2013). The profession of school nurses. In Selekman, J. (Ed.), *School nursing: A comprehensive text* (2nd ed., pp. 25–47). Philadelphia: F.A. Davis.

Zacharski, S., Minchella, L., Gomez, S., Grogan, S., Porter, S., & Robarge, D. (2013). Do not attempt resuscitation (DNAR) orders in school settings: Special needs school nurses review current research and issues. *NASN School Nurse, March,* 71–75.

Appendix A.
NASN Code of Ethics for School Nurses

Preamble

Acknowledging the diversity of the laws and conditions under which school nurses practice, the National Association of School Nurses (NASN) believes in a commonality of moral and ethical conduct. As such, NASN adopts the American Nurses Association's (ANA) *Code of Ethics for Nurses with Interpretive Statements* (2015), which establishes an ethical foundation for all nurses. Furthermore, this foundation is supported by the *School Nursing: Scope and Standards of Practice, 2nd Edition* (ANA & NASN, 2011) and ethical guidelines provided by state boards of nursing. School nursing practice, built upon these ethical foundations, is grounded in the NASN core values of child well-being, diversity, excellence, innovation, integrity, leadership, and scholarship (NASN, 2015). It is the responsibility of both the individual nurse and nursing organizations to function within these ethical provisions. For the purpose of this document the term *student* also refers to families and school communities.

Organizational Ethics

NASN, a 501(c)(3) non-profit organization established to support student health through the advancement of school nursing practice, has ethical responsibilities to its members and the communities those members serve (NASN, 2015). These organizational responsibilities include:

- Promotion of ethical work environments that support student and community health;

- Development of ". . . a research agenda that will lead to a culture of ethical practice in diverse settings that is evidence-based and measurable in terms of outcomes . . ." (Johns Hopkins School of Nursing & Johns Hopkins Berman Institute of Bioethics, 2014, p. 5);

- Development of relationships with organizations whose principles and actions are in harmony with NASN's mission and values and the termination of relationships with organizations whose known actions violate NASN's business and ethical principles; and

- Support of the role of the school nurse through advocacy, integrity, and participation in public policy development and social justice.

School Nurse Ethics

School nurses straddle two statutory and regulatory frameworks, health and education. Because school nurses practice nursing in an educationally focused system, they face unique legal, policy, funding and supervisory issues that may also have ethical dimensions. These issues may include:

- Unsafe school nurse to student ratios,
- Accountability for care delegated to Unlicensed Assistive Personnel (UAP),
- School administrator request to amend documentation,
- School administrator assignment of nursing tasks to UAP without the input of the school nurse, and
- Parent/guardian request for medical treatment for his/her student, which is inconsistent with school nurse scope of practice (Brent, 2013).

As such, school nurses must have not only the skills to communicate within both the healthcare and education arenas, but also the requisite knowledge and skills to interpret applicable laws, regulations, and professional standards, as well as apply ethical theories and principles (ANA & NASN, 2011).

Child Well-Being

- School nurses support and promote student abilities to achieve the highest quality of life as understood by each individual and family.
- School nurses integrate "caring, kindness, and respect into nursing practice" (ANA & NASN, 2011, p. 51).
- School nurses serve a unique role in transition planning to address student health needs within the school environment.
- School nurses maintain protection of, and confidentiality with, student health records according to the Health Insurance Portability and Accountability Act (HIPAA), Family Education Rights Protection Act (FERPA), other applicable federal laws, state laws and regulations, and professional standards of practice to safeguard privacy.

- School nurses utilize interventions designed to mitigate the effects of adverse childhood experiences and other social determinants of health.
- School nurses refer students to other health professionals and community health agencies as needed to promote health and well-being.

Diversity

- School nurses deliver care in a manner that promotes and preserves student autonomy, dignity, and rights so that all are treated equally regardless of race, gender, socio-economic status, culture, age, sexual orientation, gender identity, disability, or religion.
- School nurses deliver care in an inclusive, collaborative manner that embraces diversity in the school community.
- School nurses actively promote student health, safety, and self-worth.
- School nurses intervene to eliminate discrimination and bullying.

Excellence

- School nurses must have knowledge relevant to meet the needs of the student and maintain the highest level of competency by enhancing professional knowledge and skills and by collaborating with peers, other health professionals, and community agencies.
- School nurses incorporate information from supervisory clinical evaluation to improve their nursing practice.
- School nurses evaluate their own nursing practice in relation to professional standards of practice and applicable laws, regulations, and policies.

Innovation

- School nurses utilize available research in developing health programs, individual plans of care, and interventions.
- School nurse workplace environments impact the quality of health care; therefore, school nurses collaborate to improve these environments.
- School nurses are aware of social determinants of health in the school community, provide health care to all students, support school staff, and partner with families and other community members to reduce health disparities.

Integrity

- School nurses maintain confidentiality within the legal, regulatory, and ethical parameters of health and education.

- School nurses understand, follow, and inform others about student health record protection according to HIPAA, FERPA, other applicable federal laws, and state laws and regulations.

- School nurses take "appropriate action regarding instances of illegal, unethical, or inappropriate behavior that can endanger or jeopardize the best interest of the healthcare consumer or situation" (ANA & NASN, 2011, p. 50).

Leadership

- School nurses are student advocates.

- School nurses support student rights in navigating the educational environment.

- Delegation or assignment of nursing tasks, including accountability for delegated tasks, may be the responsibility of the school nurse. School nurse assignments and delegations must be consistent with state nurse practice guidelines and established best practice.

- School nurses work within educational institutions to define and implement professional standards of practice and school health policy development.

Scholarship

- School nurses are life-long learners in pursuit of knowledge, training, and experiences that enhance the quality of their nursing practice.

- School nurses participate in and promote research activities as a means of advancing student health and school health services.

- School nurses conduct research as appropriate to the nurse's education, position, and practice environment.

- School nurses adhere to the ethics that govern research, specifically:

  - Rights to privacy and confidentiality;

  - Voluntary and informed consent; and

  - Awareness of and participation in the mechanisms available to ensure the rights of human subjects, particularly vulnerable populations (e.g., minors, disabled).

Conclusion

In the course of day-to-day practice and based upon the applicable state nurse practice act and professional scope and standards of practice, school nurses may find themselves in situations that present ethical dilemmas. School nurses and school nurse organizations have a responsibility to practice in accordance with the NASN core values, *NASN Code of Ethics*, and professional standards of practice. School nurse decision-making is guided by these principles that promote improved student health, academic success, and excellence in school health services. NASN believes the practice of school nursing demands a vigilant focus on ethics.

References

American Nurses Association. (2015). *Code of ethics for nurses with interpretive statements.* Silver Spring, MD: Nursebooks.org.

American Nurses Association & National Association of School Nurses. (2011). *School nursing: Scope and standards of practice* (2nd ed.). Silver Spring, MD: Nursebooks.org.

Brent, N. (2013, July 15). *The state nurse practice act, nursing ethics and school nursing practice* [Blog post]. Retrieved from http://www.cphins.com/blog/post/the-state-nurse-practice-act-nursing-ethics-and-school-nursing-practice.

Johns Hopkins School of Nursing & Johns Hopkins Berman Institute of Bioethics. (2014, November). *A blueprint for 21st century nursing ethics: Report of the national nursing summit— Executive summary.* Retrieved from http://www.bioethicsinstitute.org/wp-content/uploads/2014/09/Executive_summary.pdf.

National Association of School Nurses. (2015, June). *About NASN.* Retrieved from https://www.nasn.org/AboutNASN.

Appendix B.
The Development of School Nursing Standards: Foundational Documents, 1900s to Present

The history of school nursing standards of practice is nearly as long as the history of the specialty itself. Publications by several individuals and organizations trace a developmental trajectory of nearly 100 years during which consensus documents about the role and functions of school nurse proved fundamental to developing future standards of practice and professional performance.

The National Association of School Nurses (NASN) has been leading the development of the standards for this specialty in recent decades. During the mid-20th century, however, other groups and individuals have played key roles in generating documents that articulated a comprehensive school nursing role. These works contributed significantly to the thinking that culminated in the development of the first set of universally endorsed standards of practice for school nursing. Some of these seminal works are listed in the following timeline. Committee chairs, authors, and editors are noted when known.

A Timeline of the Development of School Nursing Standards

1917	The first "textbook" of school nursing, *The School Nurse*, is published. Lina Rogers Struthers, the first U.S. school nurse, is the author. Struthers preceded her book with several articles on school nursing published in *The American Journal of Nursing*, one as early as 1903.
1920s–1950s	**National Organization for Public Health Nursing** (NOPHN) publishes numerous statements on the role, function, and preparation of the public health nurse in the school.
1930s–1970s	Textbooks about school nursing are published.
	1931: *School Nursing* (Mary Ella Chayer, author).
	1953: *School Nursing in the Community Program* (Marie Swanson, author).
	1963: *The Nurse in the School Health Program* (Gertrude Cromwell, author).
	1973: *School Nursing in Transition* (Doris Bryan, author).

1956	**American Public Health Association** (APHA), Committee on School Nursing, publishes *Cooperative Formulations of School Nurse Functions.*
1956, 1959	**American School Health Association** (ASHA), Committee on School Nursing Policies and Practices, publishes two editions of *Recommended Policies and Practices for School Nursing* (Eunice Lamona, Lyda Smiley, and Irma Fricke, co-committee chairs).
1955, 1961, 1966	**American Nurses Association**, School Nurses Branch, publishes three editions of *Functions, Standards, and Qualifications of School Nurses.*
1963	*Evaluation of School Nursing Activities: A Pilot Project Using a Scoring System and Accepted Standards of School Nursing* is published (Delores Basco, Supervising Public Health Nurse, Baltimore City Health Department, author).
1967	**American School Health Association** publishes *The Nurse in the School Health Program: Guidelines for School Nurses.*
1969	**National Council of School Nurse Organizations** publishes *The Unique Functions of the Professional School Nurse.*
1970	**Department of School Nurses** (DSN, later NASN) **of the National Education Association** (NEA) publishes *Standards for School Nurse Services* (Gemma Jean, committee chair).
1970–Present	**Department of School Nurses/National Association of School Nurses** publishes *School Nurse*, later *The Journal of School Nursing*, and the *NASN Newsletter*, later *NASN School Nurse*; the **American School Health Association** publishes *The Journal of School Health.*
1973	**American Nurses Association** publishes the first "generic" standards for all of nursing: *Standards of Nursing Practice* with subsequent revisions in 1991, 1998, 2004, and 2010.
1974	**American School Health Association's** School Nurse Section revises earlier work and publishes *Guidelines for the School Nurse in the School Health Program* (Virginia Thompson, committee chair).
1981	*School Nursing: A Framework for Practice* is published (Susan Wold, editor and contributing author).
1981, 1990	**National Association of School Nurses** publishes *Guidelines for the Model School Nurse Services Program* (Helen Weber, committee chair). The book was revised and updated nine years later (Susan Proctor, author).
1983	**American Nurses Association** publishes the first practice standards for school nursing developed and endorsed interorganizationally: *Standards of School Nursing Practice* (Georgia Macdonough, committee chair).

1991	**American School Health Association** publishes an implementation guide for the 1983 standards of practice: *Implementation Guide for the Standards of School Nursing Practice* (Alicia Snyder, editor and committee chair).
1993	**National Association of School Nurses** publishes an implementation guide for 1983 standards of practice: *School Nursing Practice: Roles and Standards* (Susan Proctor, author, with Susan Lordi and Donna Zaiger).
1998	**National Association of School Nurses and American Nurses Association** publish the next edition of the school nursing standards: *Standards of Professional School Nursing Practice* (Charla Dunham, committee chair).
2000	**National Association of School Nurses** publishes an implementation guide for the 1998 standards: *Standards of Professional School Nursing Practice: Applications in the Field* (Susan Lordi, author, with Beverly Bradley).
2001	**National Association of School Nurses and American Nurses Association** republish the 1998 standards with no changes but with the addition of a "scope of practice" statement: *Scope and Standards of Professional School Nursing Practice* (Charla Dunham, committee chair).
2005	**National Association of School Nurses and American Nurses Association** publish the next edition of school nursing standards: *School Nursing: Scope and Standards of Practice* (Elizabeth "Libby" Thomas, committee chair and editor).
2006, 2013	*School Nursing: A Comprehensive Text* is first published in 2006 (Janice Selekman, editor and contributing author).
2011	**National Association of School Nurses and American Nurses Association** publish *School Nursing: Scope and Standards of Practice* (2nd ed.; Elizabeth "Libby" Thomas, committee chair).
2017	**National Association of School Nurses and American Nurses Association** publish *School Nursing: Scope and Standards of Practice* (3rd ed;* Cheryl-Ann Resha, committee chair).

(* The 2017 revision, while the third edition with this title, is also the sixth iteration of a sequence of published standards: 1983; 1998; 2001; 2005; 2011; 2017.

Appendix C
School Nursing: Scope and Standards of Practice, 2nd edition, 2011

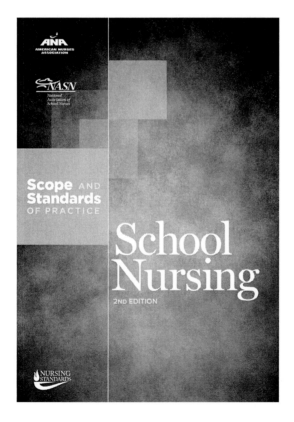

The content of the selected pages reproduced in this appendix are
not current and is of historical significance only.

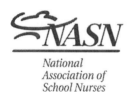

National
Association of
School Nurses

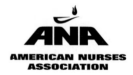

AMERICAN NURSES
ASSOCIATION

SCHOOL NURSING:
SCOPE AND STANDARDS
OF PRACTICE

nurses
books
.org
The Publishing Program of ANA

AMERICAN NURSES ASSOCIATION
SILVER SPRING, MD
2005

Appendix C. School Nursing: Scope and Standards of Practice, 2nd edition, 2011

Library of Congress Cataloging-in-Publication data

National Association of School Nurses (U.S.)
  School nursing : scope and standards of practice / National Association of School Nurses.
    p. ; cm.
  Includes bibliographical references and index.
  ISBN-13: 978-1-55810-227-9
  ISBN-10: 1-55810-227-2
  1. School nursing—Standards—United States.
  [DNLM: 1. School Nursing.   2. Nursing Process. WY 113 N277sh 2005]   I. American Nurses Association.   II. Title.

RJ247.N38 2005
371.7′12—dc22   2005014707

The American Nurses Association (ANA) is a national professional association. This ANA publication—*School Nursing: Scope and Standards of Practice*—reflects the thinking of the nursing profession on various issues and should be reviewed in conjunction with state board of nursing policies and practices. State law, rules, and regulations govern the practice of nursing, while *School Nursing: Scope and Standards of Practice* guides nurses in the application of their professional skills and responsibilities.

Published by nursesbooks.org
The Publishing Program of ANA

American Nurses Association
8515 Georgia Avenue, Suite 400
Silver Spring, MD 20910
1-800-274-4ANA
http://www.nursingworld.org/

ANA is the only full-service professional organization representing the nation's 2.7 million Registered Nurses through its 54 constituent member associations. ANA advances the nursing profession by fostering high standards of nursing practice, promoting the economic and general welfare of nurses in the workplace, projecting a positive and realistic view of nursing, and lobbying the Congress and regulatory agencies on healthcare issues affecting nurses and the public.

The National Association of School Nurses is the leading worldwide expert for school health services and is the only organization that represents school nurses and school nursing interests exclusively. Its mission is to advance the delivery of professional school health services in order to promote optimal health and learning in students, primarily through its programs and resources for its members, advocacy and public relations activities, and research support and initiatives.

ISBN 978-1-55810-228-6   05SSSN   5M   06/05

First printing June 2005.

CONTENTS

The content in this appendix is not current and is of historical significance only.

Appendix C. School Nursing: Scope and Standards of Practice, 2nd edition, 2011

ACKNOWLEDGMENTS

The National Association of School Nurses wishes to acknowledge and thank the following organizational representatives who served on a task force to review the 2001 *Scope and Standards of Professional School Nursing Practice* and suggest revisions:

Roberta Bavin, MN, CPNP, CS
National Association of Pediatric Nurses and Practitioners

Julia Muennich Cowell, PhD, RNC, FAAN
American Public Health Association

Charlotte Burt, MSN, MA, RNBC, FASHA
American School Health Association

Linda Davis-Aldritt, RN, MA, PHN
National Association of State School Nurse Consultants

Maria Klein-Rivera, RNC, MSN
National Center for School Health Nursing

The National Association of School Nurses appreciates the work of the Board of Directors on this document and the following individuals for their expertise and contributions:

Carol Boal, BGS, RN, NCSN
NASN Executive Committee, Board of Directors, Wyoming

Sandi Delack, BSN, MEd, RN, CSNT
NASN Executive Committee, Board of Directors, Rhode Island

Cynthia Galemore, BSN, MSEd, RN, NCSN
NASN Executive Committee, Kansas

Janis Hootman, RN, PhD, NCSN
NASN President, Oregon

Sally Hrymak Hunter, RN, BSN, NCSN
NASN Vice President, New Mexico

Patricia Krin, MSN, APRN, FNP, NCSN
NASN Executive Committee, Connecticut

Wanda Miller, RN, MA, NCSN, FNASN
NASN Former President and Executive Director, Colorado

The content in this appendix is not current and is of historical significance only.

Norma Nikkola, RN, BS, MS
NASN Board, Ohio

Susan Praeger, RN, EdD
School Nurse Educator, Ohio

Susanne Tullos, RN, MNSc, MSBA, NCSN
NASN Secretary, Arkansas

Susan Will, RN, MPH, NCSN, FNASN
NASN President-elect, Minnesota

Linda C. Wolfe, RN, BSN, MEd, NCSN
NASN Past President, Delaware

In addition, I wish to thank Dr. Carol Bickford, Senior Policy Fellow of the Department of Nursing Practice and Policy of the American Nurses Association, for her many suggestions and unfailing support during the review and revision process.

Elizabeth L. Thomas, RN, BS, MEd, NCSN
NASN Task Force Leader and Editor, Delaware

ANA Staff

Carol J. Bickford, PhD, RN,BC – Content editor
Yvonne Humes, MSA – Project coordinator
Winifred Carson, JD – Legal counsel

PREFACE

The contents of this document have evolved over time to frame the current role and practice of school nurses in many locales across the country and in American schools abroad. School nursing has had standards of practice since 1983, when a task force of the National Association of School Nurses, chaired by Georgia McDonough of Arizona, produced the first set of standards specific to the specialty (ANA 1983). These were modeled on early generic standards authored by the American Nurses Association (ANA). The 1983 standards served school nursing well and were the basis for the development of three implementation manuals: one by the American School Health Association (Snyder 1991), and two by the National Association of School Nurses (Proctor 1990; Proctor, Lordi, and Zaiger 1993).

The scope of practice statement describes the who, what, where, when, why, and how of school nursing practice. Review and discussion by professional school nurses focused on answering these questions and resulted in the revised scope statement. Originally written by Leslie Cooper, RN, MSN, CS, FNP, and Donna Mazyck, RN, MS, NCSN, and first published with the standards in 2001, the Scope of Practice statement has been updated and expanded, but its character remains unchanged. The standards in this document are based on the template language in *Nursing: Scope and Standards of Practice* (ANA 2004). Careful additions and substitutions make this document unique to school nursing.

The scope and standards for school nursing were approved by the National Association of School Nurses Board of Directors in November 2004 and submitted to ANA's Committee on Nursing Practice Standards and Guidelines for review. In March 2005 the ANA Congress on Nursing Practice and Economics completed its review and approved the scope of practice statement for school nursing and acknowledged the standards of practice for school nursing.

Together, the scope statement and standards describe the professional expectations of school nurses. The standards serve as a definitive guide for role implementation, interpretation, and evaluation. They are useful for the writing of position descriptions for the school nurse and for planning relevant professional development programs. The scope and standards of school nursing practice are also used in conjunction with state nurse practice acts and other relevant laws or regulations to determine the adequacy of school nursing practice. This document further defines and clarifies the role of school nurses within schools and communities.

Dr. Janis Hootman, President of the National Association of School Nurses, often has spoken of the legacy that school nurses provide for their colleagues and clients. It is with great optimism that this framework is offered to school nurses to help them channel their vast energies into health and academic achievement for all students. The legacy of high expectations for a long healthy life and lifelong learning is a gift school nurses strive to give every day to their clients.

Appendix C. School Nursing: Scope and Standards of Practice, 2nd edition, 2011

INTRODUCTION

The Standards of School Nursing Practice and their accompanying measurement criteria describe and measure a competent level of school nursing practice and professional performance. Built on ANA's *Nursing: Scope and Standards of Practice* (ANA 2004) for registered nurses, these standards are authoritative statements of the accountability, direction, and evaluation of individuals in this specialty nursing practice. Composed of two sets—the Standards of Practice and the Standards of Professional Performance—these standards define how outcomes for school nurse activities can be measured.

The Standards of Practice reflect the six steps of the nursing process (assessment, diagnosis, outcomes identification, implementation, planning, and evaluation), which is the foundation for the critical thinking of all registered nurses. The Standards of Professional Performance describe the expected behaviors expected of the nurse in the role of a school nurse.

Also included in this book is a detailed statement on the scope of school nursing practice. This discussion describes the context of this specialty practice, effectively answering the essential questions: the who, what, where, when, why, and how of school nursing practice.

Current nursing practice reflects a number of themes that underlie all nursing practice and have significant meaning for school nursing practice (ANA 2004):

- Providing age-appropriate and culturally and ethnically sensitive care
- Maintaining a safe environment
- Educating patients [clients] about healthy practices and treatment modalities
- Assuring continuity of care
- Coordinating the care across settings and among caregivers
- Managing information
- Communicating effectively
- Utilizing technology.

School nursing practice embraces and uses these themes in current practice. In fact, a communication standard was part of the *Scope and Standards of Professional School Nursing Practice* (NASN 2001). It is not a separate standard in the current publication because communication is part of each of the standards. Effective communication is still the cornerstone of the school nurse's practice.

Taken together, the contents of this book delineate the professional responsibilities of all school nurses engaged in clinical practice. This and other documents, such as position statements and issue briefs, could serve as the basis for:

- Quality improvement systems;
- Databases;
- Regulatory systems;
- Healthcare reimbursement and financial methodologies;
- Development and evaluation of nursing service delivery systems and organizational structures;
- Certification activities;
- Position descriptions and performance appraisals;
- Agency policies, procedures, and protocols; and
- Educational offerings.

Standards and practice guidelines must be evaluated regularly. School nurses are invited to provide feedback to the National Association of School Nurses regarding the usefulness, effectiveness, and comprehensiveness of this document. Keep in mind that it cannot account for all possible developments in practice. Guidelines, documents, and local protocols and procedures, as well as federal and state regulations and nurse practice acts, provide further direction.

Appendix C. School Nursing: Scope and Standards of Practice, 2nd edition, 2011

Standards of School Nursing Practice:
Standards of Practice

Standard 1. Assessment
The school nurse collects comprehensive data pertinent to the client's health or the situation.

Standard 2. Diagnosis
The school nurse analyzes the assessment data to determine the diagnosis or issues.

Standard 3. Outcomes Identification
The school nurse identifies expected outcomes for a plan individualized to the client or the situation.

Standard 4. Planning
The school nurse develops a plan that prescribes strategies and alternatives to attain expected outcomes.

Standard 5. Implementation
The school nurse implements the identified plan.

Standard 5a: Coordination of Care
The school nurse coordinates care delivery.

Standard 5b: Health Teaching and Health Promotion
The school nurse provides health education and employs strategies to promote health and a safe environment.

Standard 5c: Consultation
The school nurse provides consultation to influence the identified plan, enhance the abilities of others, and effect change.

Standard 5d: Prescriptive Authority and Treatment
The advanced practice registered nurse uses prescriptive authority, procedures, referrals, treatments, and therapies in accordance with state and federal laws and regulations.

Standard 6. Evaluation
The school nurse evaluates progress towards achievement of outcomes.

STANDARDS OF SCHOOL NURSING PRACTICE:
STANDARDS OF PROFESSIONAL PERFORMANCE

STANDARD 7. QUALITY OF PRACTICE
The school nurse systematically enhances the quality and effectiveness of nursing practice.

STANDARD 8. EDUCATION
The school nurse attains knowledge and competency that reflects current school nursing practice.

STANDARD 9. PROFESSIONAL PRACTICE EVALUATION
The school nurse evaluates one's own nursing practice in relation to professional standards and guidelines, relevant statutes, rules, and regulations.

STANDARD 10. COLLEGIALITY
The school nurse interacts with, and contributes to the professional development of, peers and school personnel as colleagues.

STANDARD 11. COLLABORATION
The school nurse collaborates with the client, the family, school staff, and others in the conduct of school nursing practice.

STANDARD 12. ETHICS
The school nurse integrates ethical provisions in all areas of practice.

STANDARD 13. RESEARCH
The school nurse integrates research findings into practice.

STANDARD 14. RESOURCE UTILIZATION
The school nurse considers factors related to safety, effectiveness, cost, and impact on practice in the planning and delivery of school nursing services.

STANDARD 15. LEADERSHIP
The school nurse provides leadership in the professional practice setting and the profession.

STANDARD 16. PROGRAM MANAGEMENT
The school nurse manages school health services.

SCOPE OF SCHOOL NURSING PRACTICE

Definitions and Distinguishing Characteristics

Nursing is the protection, promotion, and optimization of health and abilities, prevention of illness and injury, alleviation of suffering through the diagnosis and treatment of human response, and advocacy in the care of individuals, families, communities, and populations (ANA 2003a). "School Nursing is a specialized practice of professional nursing that advances the well-being, academic success, and lifelong achievement and health of students. To that end, school nurses facilitate positive student responses to normal development; promote health and safety; intervene with actual and potential health problems; provide case management services; and actively collaborate with others to build student and family capacity for adaptation, self-management, self advocacy, and learning" (NASN 1999b).

School nursing takes place primarily within local education agencies serving school-age children. However, school nurses also provide services in alternative sites (e.g., juvenile justice centers, alternative treatment centers, preschools, college campuses, learning sites for children of personnel in the armed services, and residential campuses) and within the larger surrounding community, at students' homes, vocational/occupational settings, environmental camps, field trips, school-sanctioned competitions, and sporting events.

The school nurse is likely to be the only healthcare provider in the educational setting. Unlike other healthcare workers—such as occupational therapists, physical therapists, and school psychologists, all of whom have specific defined caseloads—the school nurse is responsible for all students in a given school, district, or region. The school nurse collaborates with other health professionals to provide successful interventions for positive client outcomes. School nurses are frequently called upon to delegate nursing care to teachers, school office staff, classroom assistants, and other unlicensed assistive personnel (UAP). School nurses must be fully aware of the applicable laws, regulations, and standards pertaining to delegation of nursing tasks to others. Some states have laws or regulations prohibiting such delegation.

School nurses are most commonly employed by local school districts or education systems, although health systems such as public health, hospitals, and private health corporations may be the employer. School nurses work in a variety of delivery models such as consultant or direct services provider. They work with individuals, as well as populations, serving students from birth through age 21 or even older. The "client" of the school nurse includes not only the student, but also the student's family, the staff and faculty of the school, and the school community at large. Key roles of the school nurse include clinician, advocate, social service coordinator, health educator, liaison, and interdisciplinary student services team member (Wolfe 2005):

> Since the inception of school nursing, at the turn of the twentieth century, the specialty practice has embraced both health and education initiatives to promote the health and well-being of children. Lillian Wald, founder, envisioned a role for the school nurse to serve all, regardless of economic or social stature, or origin of nationality. She merged public health goals (to be free of communicable disease, which was of epidemic proportions), educational goals (to eliminate absenteeism from exclusion based upon contagious status), and social goals (to build literate and productive citizens). Medical goals focused on identification and exclusion of children. School nursing goals focused on inclusion.

In today's world, communicable diseases are not the only health related barriers to education. Some of the issues school nurses must address include:

- Child abuse and neglect;
- Domestic and school violence;
- Child and adolescent obesity and inactivity;
- Suicide;
- Alcohol, tobacco, and other drug use;
- Adolescent pregnancy and parenting;
- Environmental health;
- Physical and emotional disabilities and their consequences;
- Mental health;

- Children with complex physical needs; and
- Lack of health insurance coverage

School nursing is the pivotal component in continuity of care through the coordination, planning, delivery, and assessment of school health services. School nurses use the nursing process, the six steps of which—assessment, diagnosis, outcomes identification, implementation, planning, evaluation—and are the basis for the Standards of Practice. Among its other uses, this process helps to promote student and staff health and safety. School nurses also develop team relationships within the school and with community providers so that care is coordinated across settings to meet individual health needs and to avoid duplication of services.

The school nurse's primary role is to support student learning by acting as an advocate and liaison between the home, the school, and the medical community regarding concerns that may affect a student's ability to learn (NASN 1999b). Specific responsibilities are as diverse as the clients and communities served. The school nurse provides comprehensive services in all components of a coordinated school health program (Marx, Wooley, and Northrup 1998):

- Health services—Serves as the coordinator of the health services program, provides nursing care, advocates for health rights and optimization of health and abilities, and provides referral for services.
- Health education—Provides appropriate health information that promotes health and informed healthcare decisions, prevents disease, and enhances school performance.
- Environment—Identifies health and safety concerns in the school community, promotes a safe and nurturing school environment, and promotes injury prevention.
- Nutrition—Supports school food service programs and promotes the benefits of healthy eating patterns.
- Physical education and activity—Promotes healthy activities, physical education, and sports policies and practices that promote safety, good sportsmanship, and a lifelong active lifestyle.
- Counseling and mental health—Provides health counseling, assesses mental health needs, provides interventions, refers students to appropriate school staff or community agencies, and provides follow-up once treatment is prescribed.

The content in this appendix is not current and is of historical significance only.

- Parent and community involvement—Promotes community participation in assuring a healthy school and serves as school liaison to a health advisory committee.
- Staff wellness—Provides health education and counseling, and promotes healthy activities and environment for school staff.

Continuum of School Nursing Practice

School nursing exists on a continuum from the beginner through the veteran. Both the generalist school nurse and the school nurse practitioner with advanced practice training must hold current licensure as registered nurses in the state in which they practice.

Because of the complexity of issues addressed by the school nurse, the National Association of School Nurses (NASN) recommends as the minimum education for a school nurse a baccalaureate degree in nursing (BSN) from an accredited college or university, as well as state certification in states that require or recommend certification for state school nurses. Those school nurse generalists who have not acquired these credentials are strongly encouraged to aspire to and achieve these qualifications. NASN also recommends that school nurse generalists demonstrate their knowledge of school nursing by acquiring certification in the specialty of school nursing, which also requires a bachelor's degree. The NCSN credential is awarded by the National Board for Certification of School Nurses to those who pass the school nurse certification examination.

The continuum of school nurse practice includes other school nurse professionals such as advanced practice registered nurses, school nurse consultants, school nurse supervisors and administrators, lead nurses, or team leaders. There are school nurses in lead roles at school districts, regions, counties, and at the state level. As lifelong learners, school nurses seek professional development to increase critical thinking skills and professional judgment as well as to maintain current skills and knowledge. In some states, professional development is tied to licensure, but, in any case, school nurses have a professional responsibility to increase their own personal body of knowledge.

School nurses, whether generalists or advanced practice nurses, employ a community health focus in their practice. Health services are provided within the framework of primary, secondary, and tertiary prevention. Programs and services are offered with the goal of prevention—to individual students as well as to the entire school community.

School Nurse

The school nurse provides health education, health promotion, preventive health services, health assessment, and referral services to clients and staff. The actions of the school nurse focus on strengthening and facilitating students' educational outcomes, and may be directed toward individual students, family, segments of the school population, the entire school population, the school community, or the larger surrounding community. The school nurse serves as the liaison between the school, community healthcare providers, and the school-based or school-linked clinics. "As the healthcare expert within the school system, the school nurse takes a leadership role in the development and evaluation of school health policies. The school nurse participates in and provides leadership to coordinated school health programs, crisis/disaster management teams, and school health advisory councils" (NASN 2002).

The school nurse must demonstrate expertise in pediatric and adolescent health assessment, community health, and adult and child mental health nursing. Strong skills in health promotion, assessment and referral, communication, leadership, organization, and time management are essential. Knowledge of health and education laws that affect students is critical, as are teaching strategies for the delivery of health education to clients and staff, individually and collectively. School nurses are often physically isolated from other nursing and healthcare colleagues; therefore they need to be comfortable and skilled with independent management of the health office and the client caseload (Wolfe 2005).

The functions of the school nurse are to promote academic success and provide optimal nursing care to the entire school community. To these ends, the school nurse most often employs the six steps of the nursing process (adapted from ANA 2004):

- Assessment—Collects comprehensive data.

- Diagnosis—Analyzes data to determine the *nursing* diagnoses or issues.

- Outcomes identification—Identifies *measurable* expected outcomes for a plan.

- Planning—Develops a plan to attain expected outcomes.
- Implementation—Implements the plan.
- Evaluation—Evaluates progress toward attainment of outcomes.

Advanced Practice Registered Nurse

Some school nurses may meet the standards for Advanced Practice Registered Nurses (APRNs) as a result of their education, experience, skill, and authority to practice by their state licensing board. APRNs have advanced degrees and national certification in their specialty. They can be nurse practitioners or clinical specialists or both. They are differentiated by educational preparation and clinical practice. APRNs are often part of an enhanced school services team that offers health care beyond basic core services. The APRN working in the school must be knowledgeable about and competent in the standards expected of the school nurse. APRNs can offer a cost-effective solution to identified needs for students who do not receive "consistent, appropriate medical care" contributing to barriers to learning. "The anticipated outcome is more health needs of students being met, resulting in a positive impact on the health and educational performance of students" (NASN 2003).

Nursing Role Specialty

Nursing role specialties are advanced levels of nursing practice that intersect with other bodies of knowledge, have a direct influence on nursing practice, and support the delivery of direct care rendered to patients by other registered nurses. School nurses with additional professional experience and education may elect to conduct their school nursing practice within administration, education, case management, informatics, research, or other role specialties. The school nurse in a nursing role specialty should have a master's or doctoral degree. The school nurse in a role specialty is expected to comply with the standards of practice and professional performance and the associated measurement criteria for all school nurses and the additional measurement criteria for the role specialist. Other resources, such as *Scope and Standards for Nurse Administrators* (ANA 2003b), may provide additional direction.

Appendix C. School Nursing: Scope and Standards of Practice, 2nd edition, 2011

Ethical Considerations

The degree to which the school environment supports nursing practice affects the delivery of nursing care. *Healthy People 2010* cites a recommended school nurse to student ratio of 1:750 in the national health objectives (USDHHS 2000). The appropriateness of this ratio is dependent on the needs of the school population. School nurses must be able to practice nursing in an educationally focused system and clearly communicate in both the healthcare and education arenas. School nurses face unique policy, funding, and supervisory issues.

The school nurse practices in an environment that has changed dramatically since the early twentieth century. The Individuals with Disabilities Act of 1997, section 504 of the Rehabilitation Act of 1973, and the Americans with Disabilities Act of 1990 removed barriers that hindered students' access to education. Education regulations heighten the complexity of decision-making and practice, such as those of the Family Education Rights and Privacy Act (FERPA) of 1974, and subsequent amendments regarding Do Not Resuscitate orders in the school setting. The restrictions to medical information imposed by the Health Information Portability and Accessibility Act (HIPAA) of 1996 present an ongoing challenge to the school nurse who needs information about student medical needs for adequate care at school.

School nurses are advocates for their clients—students, families, school staff, and the community. They provide care to their clients that is both age-appropriate and culturally and ethnically sensitive. School nurses promote active informed participation in health decisions. They respect the individual's right to be treated with dignity, and understand the ethical and legal issues surrounding an individual's right to privacy and confidentiality. The school nurse treats all members of the school community equally, regardless of race, gender, social or economic status, culture, age, sexual orientation, disability, or religion.

The school nurse maintains the highest level of competency by enhancing professional knowledge and skills, collaborating with peers and other health professionals and community agencies, and adhering to these documents: *Nursing's Social Policy Statement* (ANA 2003a), *Code of Ethics for Nurses with Interpretive Statements* (ANA 2001), *Code of Ethics with Interpretive Statements for the School Nurse* (NASN 1999a), and the current scope and standards of school nursing. School nurses participate in the profession's efforts to advance the standards of practice, expand the body of knowledge through nursing research, and improve conditions of employment. School nurses are expected to regulate themselves; they are responsible to themselves and others for the quality of their practice. The school nurse is autonomous and must engage in considerable reflection for quality assurance.

Summary

School nurses continue to adapt their practice to a changing world. New challenges continue to present themselves, as do new tools to assist the school nurse in meeting these challenges. As technology advances, so does the school nurse's practice. Students with more complex daily health needs, as well as those requiring intermittent on-site medical treatments, are in schools across America every day. Technology is available, not only as a classroom tool and for expanded school health record keeping, but also to give students with health impairments greater access to the education to which they are entitled.

Healthy children are successful learners. The school nurse has a multi-faceted role within the school setting, one that supports the physical, emotional, mental, and social health of students and their success in the learning process (NASN 2002). The future of school nursing rests on the ability of the school nurse to successfully meet the challenges in the health and education communities.

Appendix C. School Nursing: Scope and Standards of Practice, 2nd edition, 2011

STANDARDS OF SCHOOL NURSING PRACTICE
STANDARDS OF PRACTICE

School Nursing is a specialized practice of professional nursing that advances the well-being, academic success, and lifelong achievement and health of students. To that end, school nurses facilitate positive student responses to normal development; promote health and safety; intervene with actual and potential health problems; provide case management services; and actively collaborate with others to build student and family capacity for adaptation, self-management, self-advocacy, and learning. (NASN 1999b)

STANDARD 1. ASSESSMENT
The school nurse collects comprehensive data pertinent to the client's* health or the situation.

Measurement Criteria:

The school nurse:

- Systematically compares and contrasts clinical findings with normal and abnormal variations and developmental events in forming a nursing diagnosis.

- Involves the client, family, school staff, other healthcare providers, and school community, as appropriate, in holistic data collection.

- Prioritizes data collection activities based on the client's immediate condition, or anticipated needs of the client or situation.

- Uses appropriate evidence-based assessment techniques and instruments in collecting pertinent data.

- Uses analytical models and problem-solving tools.

---

* *Client* is used in these standards to better reflect the diversity of the recipients of school nursing practice. The client can be a student, the student and family as a unit, the school population, or the school community, including faculty and staff. The focus of care may shift from individual needs to the needs of a group.

Continued ▶

- Synthesizes available data, information, and knowledge relevant to the situation to identify patterns and variances.
- Documents relevant data in a retrievable format.

Additional Measurement Criterion for the Advanced Practice Registered Nurse:

The advanced practice registered nurse:

- Initiates and interprets diagnostic tests and procedures relevant to the client's current status.

Appendix C. School Nursing: Scope and Standards of Practice, 2nd edition, 2011

Standard 2. Diagnosis
The school nurse analyzes the assessment data to determine the diagnoses or issues.

Measurement Criteria:

The school nurse:

- Derives the nursing diagnoses or issues based on assessment data.
- Validates the nursing diagnoses or issues with the client, family, school staff, school community, and other healthcare providers when possible and appropriate.
- Documents nursing diagnoses or issues in a manner that facilitates the determination of the expected outcomes and plan.
- Uses standardized language or recognized terminology to document the nursing diagnosis in a retrievable form.

Additional Measurement Criteria for the Advanced Practice Registered Nurse:

The advanced practice registered nurse:

- Systematically compares and contrasts clinical findings with normal and abnormal variations and developmental events in formulating a differential diagnosis.
- Utilizes complex data and information obtained during interview, examination, and diagnostic procedures in identifying diagnoses.
- Assists staff in developing and maintaining competency in the diagnostic process.

STANDARD 3. OUTCOMES IDENTIFICATION
The school nurse identifies expected outcomes for a plan individualized to the client or the situation.

Measurement Criteria:

The school nurse:

- Involves the client, family, school staff, and other healthcare providers in formulating expected outcomes when possible and appropriate.
- Derives culturally appropriate expected outcomes from the diagnoses.
- Considers associated risks, benefits, costs, current scientific evidence, and clinical expertise when formulating expected outcomes.
- Defines expected outcomes in terms of the client, client values, ethical considerations, environment, or situation with such consideration as associated risks, benefits and costs, and current scientific evidence.
- Includes a time estimate for attainment of expected outcomes.
- Develops expected outcomes that provide direction for continuity of care.
- Modifies expected outcomes based on changes in the status of the client or evaluation of the situation.
- Documents expected outcomes as measurable goals.
- Uses standardized language or recognized terminology to document the outcome in a retrievable form.

Additional Measurement Criteria for the Advanced Practice Registered Nurse:

The advanced practice registered nurse:

- Identifies expected outcomes that incorporate scientific evidence and are achievable through implementation of evidence-based practices.

Appendix C. School Nursing: Scope and Standards of Practice, 2nd edition, 2011

- Identifies expected outcomes that incorporate cost and clinical effectiveness, client satisfaction, and continuity and consistency among providers.
- Supports the use of clinical guidelines linked to positive client outcomes.

STANDARD 4. PLANNING
The school nurse develops a plan that prescribes strategies and alternatives to attain expected outcomes.

Measurement Criteria:

The school nurse:

- Develops an individualized healthcare plan considering the client characteristics or the situation (e.g., age and culturally appropriate, environmentally sensitive), with appropriate strategies for health promotion and disease prevention.

- Develops the plan in conjunction with the client, family, school community, and others, as appropriate.

- Creates individual healthcare plans as a component of the program for clients with special healthcare needs.

- Provides for continuity within the plan.

- Incorporates an implementation pathway or timeline within the plan.

- Establishes the plan priorities with the client, family, school community, and others as appropriate.

- Utilizes the plan to provide direction to other members of the school team.

- Defines the plan to reflect current statutes, rules and regulations, and standards.

- Integrates current trends and research affecting care in the planning process.

- Considers the economic impact of the plan.

- Uses standardized language or recognized terminology to document the plan in a retrievable form.

Additional Measurement Criteria for the Advanced Practice Registered Nurse:

The advanced practice registered nurse:

- Identifies assessment, diagnostic strategies, and therapeutic interventions within the plan that reflect current evidence, including data, research, literature, and expert clinical knowledge.

Appendix C. School Nursing: Scope and Standards of Practice, 2nd edition, 2011

- Selects or designs strategies to meet the multifaceted needs of complex clients.
- Includes the synthesis of client's values and beliefs regarding nursing and medical therapies within the plan.

Additional Measurement Criteria for the Nursing Role Specialty:

The school nurse in a nursing role specialty:

- Participates in the design and development of multidisciplinary and interdisciplinary processes to address the situation or issue.
- Contributes to the development and continuous improvement of organizational systems that support the planning process.
- Supports the integration of clinical, human, and financial resources to enhance and complete the decision-making processes.

STANDARD 5. IMPLEMENTATION
The school nurse implements the identified plan.

Measurement Criteria:

The school nurse:

- Implements the plan in a safe and timely manner.
- Documents implementation and any modifications, including changes or omissions, of the specified plan.
- Utilizes evidence-based interventions and treatments specific to the diagnosis or problem.
- Utilizes community resources and systems to implement the plan.
- Collaborates with nursing colleagues and others to implement the plan.
- Provides interventions in compliance with these standards of practice and professional performance.
- Uses standardized language or recognized terminology to document implementation of the plan in a retrievable form.

Additional Measurement Criteria for the Advanced Practice Registered Nurse:

The advanced practice registered nurse:

- Facilitates utilization of systems and community resources to implement the plan.
- Supports collaboration with school nursing colleagues and other nursing colleagues and disciplines to implement the plan.
- Incorporates new knowledge and strategies to initiate change in school nursing care practices if desired outcomes are not achieved.

Additional Measurement Criteria for the Nursing Role Specialty:

The school nurse in a nursing role specialty:

- Implements the plan using principles and concepts of project or systems management.
- Fosters organizational systems that support implementation of the plan.

STANDARD 5A: COORDINATION OF CARE
The school nurse coordinates care delivery.

Measurement Criteria:

The school nurse:

- Coordinates creation and implementation of the individual health-care plan.
- Documents the coordination of the care.

Measurement Criteria for the Advanced Practice Registered Nurse:

The advanced practice registered nurse:

- Provides leadership in the coordination of multidisciplinary health care for integrated delivery of client care services.
- Synthesizes data and information to prescribe necessary education and healthcare system and community support measures, including environmental modifications.
- Coordinates education and healthcare system and community resources that enhance delivery of care across continuums.

STANDARD 5B: HEALTH TEACHING AND HEALTH PROMOTION
The school nurse provides health education and employs strategies to promote health and a safe environment.

Measurement Criteria:

The school nurse:

- Provides general health education to the student body at large through direct classroom instruction or expert consultation.

- Provides health teaching that addresses such topics as healthy lifestyles, risk-reducing behaviors, developmental needs, activities of daily living, and preventive self-care as appropriate to client developmental levels.

- Uses health promotion and health teaching methods appropriate to the situation and the client's developmental level, learning needs, readiness, ability to learn, language preference, and culture.

- Promotes self-care and safety through the education of the school community regarding health issues.*

- Promotes health principles through the coordinated school health program for all in the school community.

- Seeks opportunities for feedback and evaluation of the effectiveness of the strategies used.

- Participates in the assessment of needs for health education and health instruction for the school community.*

- Provides individual and group health teaching and counseling for and with clients.*

- Participates in the design and development of health education materials, and other health education activities.*

- Participates in the evaluation of health curricula and health instructional materials and activities.*

- Acts as a primary resource person to school staff (and others as appropriate) regarding health education and health education materials.*

---

*Adapted from Proctor, Lordi, and Zaiger 1993 and NASN and ANA 2001.

Appendix C. School Nursing: Scope and Standards of Practice, 2nd edition, 2011

Additional Measurement Criteria for the Advanced Practice Registered Nurse:

The advanced practice registered nurse:

- Synthesizes empirical evidence on risk behaviors, learning theories, behavioral change theories, motivational theories, epidemiology, and other related theories and frameworks when designing health information and client education.

- Designs health information and client education appropriate to the client's developmental level, learning needs, readiness to learn, and cultural values and beliefs.

- Evaluates health information resources, such as the Internet, within the area of practice for accuracy, readability, and comprehensibility to help client's access quality health information.

STANDARD 5C: CONSULTATION

The school nurse provides consultation to influence the identified plan, enhance the abilities of others, and effect change.

Measurement Criteria:

The school nurse:

- Synthesizes data, information, theoretical frameworks, and evidence when providing consultation.

- Facilitates the effectiveness of a consultation by involving the stakeholders in the decision-making process.

- Communicates consultation recommendations that influence the identified plan, facilitate understanding by involved stakeholders, enhance the work of others, and effect change.

Measurement Criteria for the Advanced Practice Registered Nurse:

The advanced practice registered nurse:

- Synthesizes clinical data, theoretical frameworks, and evidence when providing consultation.

- Facilitates the effectiveness of a consultation by involving the client when appropriate in decision-making and negotiating role responsibilities.

- Communicates consultation recommendations that facilitate change.

Appendix C. *School Nursing: Scope and Standards of Practice, 2nd edition, 2011*

STANDARD 5D: PRESCRIPTIVE AUTHORITY AND TREATMENT
The advanced practice registered nurse uses prescriptive authority, procedures, referrals, treatments, and therapies in accordance with state and federal laws and regulations.

Measurement Criteria for the Advanced Practice Registered Nurse:

The advanced practice registered nurse:

- Prescribes evidence-based treatments, therapies, and procedures considering the client's comprehensive healthcare needs.

- Prescribes pharmacologic agents based on a current knowledge of pharmacology and physiology.

- Prescribes specific pharmacological agents and/or treatments based on clinical indicators, the client's status and needs, and the results of diagnostic and laboratory tests.

- Evaluates therapeutic and potential adverse effects of pharmacological and non-pharmacological treatments.

- Provides client and family with information about intended effects and potential adverse effects of proposed prescriptive therapies.

- Provides information about costs, and alternative treatments and procedures, as appropriate.

STANDARD **6.** EVALUATION

The school nurse evaluates progress towards attainment of outcomes.

Measurement Criteria:

The school nurse:

- Conducts a systematic, ongoing, and criterion-based evaluation of the outcomes in relation to the structures and processes prescribed by the plan and the indicated timeline.

- Includes the client and others involved in the care or situation in the evaluative process.

- Evaluates the effectiveness of the planned strategies in relation to client responses and the attainment of the expected outcomes.

- Documents the results of the evaluation.

- Uses ongoing assessment data to revise the diagnoses, the outcomes, the plan, and the implementation as needed.

- Disseminates the results to the client and others involved in the care or situation, as appropriate, in accordance with client and parent directions, and state and federal laws and regulations.

Additional Measurement Criteria for the Advanced Practice Registered Nurse:

The advanced practice registered nurse:

- Evaluates the accuracy of the diagnosis and effectiveness of the interventions in relationship to the patient's attainment of expected outcomes.

- Synthesizes the results of the evaluation analyses to determine the impact of the plan on the affected clients, families, groups, communities, and institutions.

- Uses the results of the evaluation analyses to make or recommend process or structural changes, including policy, procedure, or protocol documentation, as appropriate.

Appendix C. School Nursing: Scope and Standards of Practice, 2nd edition, 2011

Additional Measurement Criteria for the Nursing Role Specialty:

The school nurse in a nursing role specialty:

- Uses the results of the evaluation analyses to make or recommend process or structural changes, including policy, procedure, or protocol documentation, as appropriate.
- Synthesizes the results of the evaluation analyses to determine the impact of the plan on the affected clients, families, groups, school communities, and institutions, networks, and organizations.

STANDARDS OF PROFESSIONAL PERFORMANCE

STANDARD 7. QUALITY OF PRACTICE
The school nurse systematically enhances the quality and effectiveness of nursing practice.

Measurement Criteria:

The school nurse:

- Demonstrates quality by documenting the application of the nursing process in a responsible, accountable, and ethical manner.

- Uses the results of quality improvement activities to initiate changes in school nursing practice and in the healthcare delivery system.

- Uses creativity and innovation in school nursing practice to improve care delivery.

- Incorporates new knowledge to initiate changes in school nursing practice if desired outcomes are not achieved.

- Participates in quality improvement activities. Such activities may include:

  - Identifying aspects of practice important for quality monitoring.

  - Using indicators developed to monitor quality and effectiveness of nursing practice.

  - Collecting data to monitor quality and effectiveness of school nursing practice.

  - Analyzing quality data to identify opportunities for improving school nursing practice.

  - Formulating recommendations to improve school nursing practice or outcomes.

  - Implementing activities to enhance the quality of school nursing practice.

Continued ▶

- Developing, implementing, and evaluating policies, procedures and/or guidelines to improve the quality of school nursing practice.
- Participating on interdisciplinary teams to evaluate clinical care or health services.
- Participating in efforts to minimize costs and unnecessary duplication.
- Analyzing factors related to safety, satisfaction, effectiveness, and cost–benefit options.
- Analyzing organizational systems for barriers.
- Obtaining and maintaining national certification in school nursing as well as state certification (if available).
- Implementing processes to remove or decrease barriers within organizational systems.

Additional Measurement Criteria for the Advanced Practice Registered Nurse:
The advanced practice registered nurse:

- Obtains and maintains professional certification if available in the area of expertise.
- Designs quality improvement initiatives.
- Implements initiatives to evaluate the need for change.
- Evaluates the practice environment and quality of nursing care rendered in relation to existing evidence, identifying opportunities for the generation and use of research.

Additional Measurement Criteria for the Nursing Role Specialty:
The school nurse in a nursing role specialty:

- Obtains and maintains professional certification if available in the area of expertise.
- Designs quality improvement initiatives.
- Implements initiatives to evaluate the need for change.
- Evaluates the practice environment in relation to existing evidence, identifying opportunities for the generation and use of research.

STANDARD **8.** EDUCATION

The school nurse attains knowledge and competency that reflects current school nursing practice.

Measurement Criteria:

The school nurse:

- Participates in ongoing educational activities related to appropriate knowledge bases and professional issues.

- Demonstrates a commitment to lifelong learning through self-reflection and inquiry to identify learning needs.

- Seeks experiences that reflect current practice in order to maintain skills and competence in clinical practice or role performance.

- Acquires knowledge and skills appropriate to the specialty area, practice setting, role, or situation.

- Maintains professional records that provide evidence of competency and lifelong learning.

- Seeks experiences and formal and independent learning activities to maintain and develop clinical and professional skills and knowledge.

Additional Measurement Criterion for the Advanced Practice Registered Nurse:

The advanced practice registered nurse:

- Uses current healthcare research findings and other evidence to expand clinical knowledge, enhance role performance, and increase knowledge of professional issues.

Additional Measurement Criterion for the Nursing Role Specialty:

The school nurse in a nursing role specialty:

- Uses current research findings and other evidence to expand knowledge, enhance role performance, and increase knowledge of professional issues.

STANDARD 9. PROFESSIONAL PRACTICE EVALUATION

The school nurse evaluates one's own nursing practice in relation to professional practice standards and guidelines, relevant statutes, rules, and regulations.

Measurement Criteria:

- The school nurse's practice reflects the application of knowledge of current practice standards, guidelines, statutes, rules, and regulations.

- The school nurse:

  - Provides age-appropriate care in a culturally and ethnically sensitive manner.

  - Engages in self-evaluation of practice on a regular basis, identifying areas of strength as well as areas in which professional development would be beneficial.

  - Obtains informal feedback regarding one's own practice from clients, peers, professional colleagues, and others.

  - Participates in systematic peer review as appropriate.

  - Takes action to achieve goals identified during the evaluation process.

  - Provides rationales for practice beliefs, decisions, and actions as part of the informal and formal evaluation processes.

Additional Measurement Criterion for the Advanced Practice Registered Nurse:

The advanced practice registered nurse:

- Engages in a formal process seeking feedback regarding one's own practice from clients, peers, professional colleagues, and others.

Additional Measurement Criterion for the Nursing Role Specialty:

The school nurse in a nursing role specialty:

- Engages in a formal process seeking feedback regarding role performance from individuals, professional colleagues, representatives and administrators of corporate entities, and others.

STANDARD 10. COLLEGIALITY
The school nurse interacts with, and contributes to the professional development of, peers and school personnel as colleagues.

Measurement Criteria:

The school nurse:

- Shares knowledge and skills with peers and colleagues as evidenced by such activities as multidisciplinary student assistance conferences or presentations at formal or informal meetings.
- Provides peers with feedback regarding their practice or role performance.
- Interacts with peers and colleagues to enhance one's own professional nursing practice and role performance and the health care of the school community.
- Maintains compassionate and caring relationships with peers and colleagues.
- Contributes to an environment that is conducive to the education of healthcare professionals and the whole school community.
- Contributes to a supportive and healthy work environment.
- Participates in appropriate professional organizations in a membership or leadership capacity.

Additional Measurement Criteria for the Advanced Practice Registered Nurse:

The advanced practice registered nurse:

- Models expert practice to interdisciplinary team members and healthcare consumers.
- Mentors other registered nurses and colleagues as appropriate.
- Participates with interdisciplinary teams that contribute to role development and advanced nursing practice and health care.

Continued ▶

Additional Measurement Criteria for the Nursing Role Specialty:

The school nurse in a nursing role specialty:

- Participates on multi-professional teams that contribute to role development and, directly or indirectly, advance nursing practice and health services.

- Mentors other registered nurses and colleagues as appropriate.

STANDARD **11.** COLLABORATION
The school nurse collaborates with the client, the family, school staff, and others in the conduct of school nursing practice.

Measurement Criteria:

The school nurse:

- Communicates with the client, the family, and healthcare providers regarding client care and the school nurse's role in the delivery of that care.
- Collaborates in creating a documented healthcare plan that is focused on outcomes and decisions related to care and delivery of services and indicates communication with clients, families, and others.
- Partners with others to effect change and generate positive outcomes through knowledge of the client or situation.
- Documents referrals, including provisions for continuity of care.

Additional Measurement Criteria for the Advanced Practice Registered Nurse:

The advanced practice registered nurse:

- Partners with other disciplines to enhance patient care through interdisciplinary activities, such as education, consultation, management, technological development, or research opportunities.
- Facilitates an interdisciplinary process with other members of the healthcare team.
- Documents plan-of-care communications, rationales for plan-of-care changes, and collaborative discussions to improve patient care.

Additional Measurement Criteria for the Nursing Role Specialty:

The school nurse in a nursing role specialty:

- Partners with others to enhance health care, and ultimately client care, through interdisciplinary activities such as education, consultation, management, technological development, or research.
- Documents plans, communications, rationales for plan changes, and collaborative discussions.

Appendix C. School Nursing: Scope and Standards of Practice, 2nd edition, 2011

STANDARD 12. ETHICS
The school nurse integrates ethical provisions in all areas of practice.

Measurement Criteria:

The school nurse:

- Uses *Code of Ethics for Nurses with Interpretive Statements* (ANA 2001) and *Code of Ethics with Interpretive Statements for School Nurses* (NASN 1999a) to guide practice.
- Delivers care in a manner that preserves and protects client autonomy, dignity, and rights, sensitive to diversity in the school setting.
- Maintains client confidentiality within legal and regulatory parameters of both health and education.
- Serves as a client advocate assisting clients in developing skills for self-advocacy.
- Maintains a therapeutic and professional client–nurse relationship with appropriate professional role boundaries.
- Demonstrates a commitment to practicing self-care, managing stress, and connecting with self and others.
- Contributes to resolving ethical issues of clients, colleagues, or systems as evidenced in such activities as participating on ethics committees.
- Reports illegal, incompetent, or impaired practices.
- Seeks available resources to formulate ethical decisions.

Additional Measurement Criteria for the Advanced Practice Registered Nurse:

The advanced practice registered nurse:

- Informs the client of the risks, benefits, and outcomes of healthcare regimens.
- Participates in interdisciplinary teams that address ethical risks, benefits, and outcomes.

Additional Measurement Criteria for the Nursing Role Specialty:

The school nurse in a nursing role specialty:

- Participates on multidisciplinary and interdisciplinary teams that address ethical risks, benefits, and outcomes.
- Informs administrators or others of the risks, benefits, and outcomes of programs and decisions that affect healthcare delivery.

STANDARD 13. RESEARCH
The school nurse integrates research findings into practice.

Measurement Criteria:

The school nurse:

- Utilizes the best available evidence, including research findings, to guide practice decisions.
- Actively participates in research activities at various levels appropriate to the school nurse's education and position. Such activities may include:
  - Identifying clinical problems specific to nursing research (client care and nursing practice).
  - Participating in data collection (surveys, pilot projects, formal studies).
  - Participating in a formal committee or program.
  - Sharing research activities or findings with peers and others.
  - Conducting research.
  - Critically analyzing and interpreting research for application to practice.
  - Using research findings in the development of policies, procedures, and standards of practice in client care.
  - Incorporating research as a basis for learning.
  - Contributing to school nursing literature.

Additional Measurement Criteria for the Advanced Practice Registered Nurse:

The advanced practice registered nurse:

- Contributes to nursing knowledge by conducting or synthesizing research that discovers, examines, and evaluates knowledge, theories, criteria, and creative approaches to improve healthcare practice.
- Formally disseminates research findings through activities such as presentations, publications, consultation, and journal clubs.

Additional Measurement Criteria for the Nursing Role Specialty:

The school nurse in a nursing role specialty:

- Contributes to nursing knowledge by conducting or synthesizing research that discovers, examines, and evaluates knowledge, theories, criteria, and creative approaches to improve health care.
- Formally disseminates research findings through activities such as presentations, publications, consultation, and journal clubs.

Standard 14. Resource Utilization

The school nurse considers factors related to safety, effectiveness, cost, and impact on practice in the planning and delivery of school nursing services.

Measurement Criteria:

The school nurse:

- Evaluates factors such as safety, effectiveness, availability, cost and benefits, efficiencies, and impact on practice, when choosing among practice options that would result in the same expected outcome.

- Assists the client and family in identifying and securing appropriate and available services to address health-related needs.

- Assigns or delegates tasks, based on the needs and condition of the client, potential for harm, stability of the client's condition, complexity of the task, and predictability of the outcome; as defined and permitted by individual state nurse practice acts; and according to the knowledge and skills of the designated caregiver.

- Assists the client and school community in becoming informed consumers about the options, costs, risks, and benefits of health promotion, health education, school health services, and individualized health interventions for clients.

Additional Measurement Criteria for the Advanced Practice Registered Nurse:

The advanced practice registered nurse:

- Utilizes organizational and community resources to formulate multidisciplinary or interdisciplinary plans of care.

- Develops innovative solutions for client care problems that address effective resource utilization and maintenance of quality.

- Develops evaluation strategies to demonstrate cost effectiveness, cost–benefit, and efficiency factors associated with nursing practice.

Additional Measurement Criteria for the Nursing Role Specialty:

The school nurse in a nursing role specialty:

- Develops innovative solutions and applies strategies to obtain appropriate resources for nursing initiatives.

- Secures organizational resources to ensure a work environment conducive to completing the identified plan and outcomes.
- Develops evaluation methods to measure safety and effectiveness for interventions and outcomes.
- Promotes activities that assist others, as appropriate, in becoming informed about costs, risks, and benefits of care or of the plan and solution.

STANDARD **15.** LEADERSHIP
The school nurse provides leadership in the professional practice setting and the profession.

Measurement Criteria:

The school nurse:

- Engages in teamwork as a team player and a team builder.

- Works to create and maintain healthy work environments in local, regional, national, or international communities.

- Displays the ability to define a clear vision, the associated goals, and a plan to implement and measure progress

- Demonstrates a commitment to continuous, lifelong learning for self and others.

- Teaches others to succeed by mentoring and other strategies.

- Exhibits creativity and flexibility through times of change.

- Demonstrates energy, excitement, and a passion for quality work.

- Willingly accepts mistakes by self and others, thereby creating a culture in which risk-taking is not only safe, but also expected.

- Inspires loyalty by valuing people as the most precious asset in an organization.

- Directs the coordination of care across settings and among care-givers, including oversight of licensed and unlicensed personnel in any assigned or delegated tasks as permitted by state nurse practice acts.

- Serves in key roles in the school and work settings by participating on committees, councils, and administrative teams.

- Promotes advancement of the profession through participation in professional school nursing and school health organizations.

- Demonstrates knowledge of the philosophy and mission of the school district, the nature of its curricular and extracurricular activities, and its programs and special services.*

---

*Adapted from Proctor, Lordi, and Zaiger 1993.

- Demonstrates knowledge of the roles of other school professionals and adjunct personnel.*
- Coordinates roles and responsibilities of the adjunct school health personnel within the school team.*

Additional Measurement Criteria for the Advanced Practice Registered Nurse:

The advanced practice registered nurse:

- Works to influence decision-making bodies to improve client care.
- Provides direction to enhance the effectiveness of the healthcare team.
- Initiates and revises protocols or guidelines to reflect evidence-based practice, to reflect accepted changes in care management, or to address emerging problems.
- Promotes communication of information and advancement of the profession through writing, publishing, and presentations for professional or lay audiences.
- Designs innovations to effect change in practice and improve health outcomes.

Additional Measurement Criteria for the Nursing Role Specialty:

The school nurse in a nursing role specialty:

- Works to influence decision-making bodies to improve client care, health services, and policies.
- Promotes communication of information and advancement of the profession through writing, publishing, and presentations for professional or lay audiences.
- Designs innovations to effect change in practice and outcomes.
- Provides direction to enhance the effectiveness of the multidisciplinary or interdisciplinary team.

Appendix C. School Nursing: Scope and Standards of Practice, 2nd edition, 2011

STANDARD 16. PROGRAM MANAGEMENT
The school nurse manages school health services.

Measurement Criteria:

The school nurse:

- Manages school health services as appropriate to the nurse's education, position, and practice environment.*

- Conducts school health needs assessments to identify current health problems and identify the need for new programs.*

- Develops and implements needed health programs using a program planning process.*

- Demonstrates knowledge of existing school health programs and current health trends that may affect client care, the sources of funds for each, school policy related to each, and local, state, and federal laws governing each.*

- **Develops and implements health policies and procedures in collaboration with the school administration, the board of health, and the board of education.***

- Evaluates ongoing health programs for outcomes and quality of care, and communicates findings to administrators and the board of education.*

- Orients, trains, documents competency, supervises, and evaluates health assistants, aides, and UAPs (unlicensed assistive personnel), as appropriate to the school setting.*

- Initiates changes throughout the healthcare delivery system, as appropriate, using the results of school health environmental needs assessments, analysis of evaluation data, and quality-of-care activities.*

- Participates in environmental safety and health activities (e.g., indoor air quality, injury surveillance and prevention).*

- Adopts and uses available technology appropriate to the work setting.*

---

*Adapted from Proctor, Lordi, and Zaiger 1993.

Glossary

Client. Recipient of (school) nursing practice (ANA 2004). The client can be a student, the student and family as a unit, the school population, or the school community (faculty and staff). The focus of care may shift from individual needs to the needs of a group.

Plan. A comprehensive outline of components of care to be delivered to attain expected outcomes (ANA 2004). This would include an individualized healthcare plan (IHP), an individualized education plan (IEP) as part of the special education regulations (IDEA), a 504 plan, and others.

Role specialty. A practice in which the school nurse primarily works in education, case management, health education, prevention (such as adolescent pregnancy and parenting, or infectious disease), program implementation (such as special education or 504 plan creation and implementation), disease specialization (such as diabetes, asthma, or cystic fibrosis), administration, or leadership (such as lead nurse or co-ordinator for a large school district). This practice requires advanced study at the master's or doctoral level and considerable expertise.

School community. All those who study and work in a school district. This could be expanded when appropriate to community agencies, faith-based groups, student families, and others.

Appendix C. School Nursing: Scope and Standards of Practice, 2nd edition, 2011

REFERENCES

American Nurses Association (ANA). 1983. Standards for professional nursing education. Kansas City, MO: ANA.

———. 2001. *Code of ethics for nurses with interpretive statements.* Washington, DC: American Nurses Publishing.

———. 2003. *Nursing's social policy statement.* 2nd Edition. Washington, DC: Nursebooks.org.

———. 2003. *Scope and standards for nurse administrators.* 2nd Edition. Washington, DC: Nursebooks.org.

———. 2004. *Nursing: Scope and standards of practice.* Washington, DC: Nursebooks.org.

Marx, E., S. Wooley, and D. Northrup, eds. 1998. *Health is academic: A guide to coordinated school health programs.* New York: Teacher's College Press.

National Association of School Nurses (NASN). 1999a. *Code of ethics with interpretive statements for school nurses.* Scarborough, ME: NASN.

———. 1999b. Definition of school nursing. Adopted at Board of Directors Meeting, June, Providence, RI.

——— and American Nurses Association (ANA). 2001. *Scope and standards of professional school nursing practice.* Washington, DC: American Nurses Publishing.

———. 2002. *Issue brief: School health nursing services role in health care.* Scarborough, ME: NASN.

———. 2003. *Position statement: Role of advanced nurse practitioner in the school setting.* Scarborough, ME: NASN.

Proctor, S.T. 1990. *Guidelines for a model school nurse services program.* Scarborough, ME: NASN.

Proctor, S.T., S.L. Lordi, and D.S. Zaiger. 1993. *School nursing practice: Roles and standards.* Scarborough, ME: NASN.

Synder, A. (ed.). 1991. *Implementation guide for the standards of school nursing practice.* Kent, OH: American School Health Association.

U.S. Department of Health and Human Services (USDHHS). 2000. *Healthy people 2010: Health objectives for the nation.* Washington, DC: USDHHS.

Wolfe, L. 2005. Roles of the school nurse. In *School nursing: A comprehensive text,* ed. J. Selekman. Philadelphia: F.A. Davis.

Index

Note: Entries with [2005] indicate an entry from *School Nursing: Scope and Standards of Practice, 2nd Edition* (2011) reproduced in this current edition as Appendix C. That information is not current' it is included for reference and historical context.

requirements for, 29
research competencies
    measurement criteria, 154
resource utilization competencies,
    81
    measurement criteria, 156
role of, 29–30
Advocacy in school nursing practice,
    21
Aggregate
    definition, 87
American Academy of Pediatrics, 24
American Association of Critical-Care
    Nurses, 23
ANA *Code of Ethics for Nurses with
Interpretive Statements*, 13
Art of school nursing, 15–16
Assessment in school nursing practice
    competencies involving, 43–45
    definition, 87
    standard of practice, 7, 43–45
    [2011], 130
Assessment data in school nursing
    practice, 2
    in diagnosis, 45–47
    in evaluation, 57
Autonomy
    definition, 87

B

Baccalaureate degree in nursing, 3
Bachelor of science in nursing (BSN), 3,
    27, 30
Bus transportation, 22

C

Care coordination, 1–2, 10, 12, 13, 16;
    s*ee also* Coordination of care
Centers for Disease Control and
    Prevention (CDC), 18
Client
    definition, 161
Coaching
    definition, 87
Code of ethics (nursing)
    definition, 87

Code of Ethics for Nurses with
    Interpretive Statements and school
    nursing practice, 13, 33–37, 99;
    see also NASN Code of Ethics for
    School Nurses
accountability and responsibility for
    practice (Provision 4), 35
advocacy for the patient (Provision 3),
    34–35
collaboration with the pubic and
    health professionals (Provision 8),
    36–37
commitment to the patient
    (Provision 2), 34
competencies involving, 62, 79
duties to self and others (Provision 5),
    35
nursing profession advancement
    (Provision 7), 36
nursing professional integrity
    and values and social justice
    (Provision 9), 37
respect for the individual (Provision 1),
    33–34
work settings and care environment
    contributions (Provision 6), 36
Collaboration in school nursing practice
    competencies involving, 68–69
    definition, 88
    standard of professional performance,
    68–69,
    [2011], 151; *see also* Care
    coordination; Coordination
    of care; Interprofessional
    collaboration
Collegiality in school nursing practice
    [2011], 121, 149–150
Communication in school nursing
    practice
    competencies involving, 66–67
    standard of professional performance,
    9, 66–67
Community health in school nursing
    practice, 14, 15
Community health nursing, 10
Community in school nursing practice,
    20, 125

Competence in school nursing practice
definition, 88
evaluation, 32–33
professional, in school nursing practice,
31–32
Competencies for school nursing standards
assessment, 43–45
collaboration, 68–69
communication, 66–67
coordination of care, 55–56
culturally congruent practice, 63–65
diagnosis, 46–47
education, 72–73
environmental health, 82–83
ethics, 61–62
evaluation, 59–60
evidence-based practice and research,
74–75
health teaching and health promotion,
57–58
implementation, 52–54
leadership, 70–71
outcomes identification, 48–49
planning, 50–51
professional practice evaluation, 79
program management, 84–86
quality of practice, 76–78
resource utilization, 80–81
Complexity
definition, 88
Confidentiality and privacy in school
nursing practice, 33, 34
Consultation in school nursing practice
[2011], 120, 141
Coordination of care in school nursing
practice [2011], 16
competencies involving, 55–56
standard of practice for, 8, 55–56, 138
Counseling in school nursing practice, 19
Crisis management plan
definition, 88
Culturally congruent practice
competencies involving, 63–65
standards of professional performance,
63–65
Culture of health
definition, 88

D

Delegation
definition, 88
Department of Defense Education
Activity (DoDEA), 3
Developmentally appropriate learning in
school nursing practice, 19
Diagnosis in school nursing practice
competencies involving, 46–47
definition, 88
standard of practice for, 7, 46–47,
132

E

Education in school nursing practice
competencies involving, 72–73
standards of professional performance,
9, 72–73, 147
Emergency action plan (EAP)
definition, 88
Emergency care plan (ECP)
definition, 88
Employee wellness, 19
Enculturation
definition, 88
Environmental health in school nursing
practice, 26
competencies involving, 82–83
standards of professional performance,
9, 82–83
Ethics in school nursing practice;
see also Code of Ethics for Nurses
with Interpretive Statements;
NASN Code of Ethics for School
Nurses
competencies involving, 62–63
ethical challenges, 37
ethical considerations, 33
standard of professional performance,
8, 61–62
Evaluation in school nursing practice
competencies involving, 59–60
definition, 89
standards of practice for, 8, 59–60
Evidence-based practice
definition, 89

S

School
  definition, 92
School community
  definition, 92, 161
School nurse [2011], 123, 126
  role of, 10
School nurse administrator
  definition, 92
School nursing
  definition, 10, 92
School nursing settings, *see* Where of
    school nursing
School Nursing Standards development,
    timeline of, 105–107
*School Nursing: Scope and Standards of
    Practice*, 5
School-based health centers (SBHC),
    21–22
Science of school nursing, 14–15
Scope of school nursing practice
  definition, 1, 92
  description of scope of school nursing
      practice, 2–4
  distinguishing characteristics, 1–2
  how of school nursing, 13–20
  professional school nurses, 27–33
  Standards of Professional Performance
      for School Nursing, 8–9
  standards of school nursing practice,
      4–8
  trends and issues in, 38–39
  what of school nursing, 10–11
  when school nursing, 25–27
  where of school nursing, 20–25
  who of school nursing, 27–33
  why of school nursing, 33–37
Scope of School Nursing Practice [2011]
  continuum of, 125–127
  definitions, 122
  distinguishing characteristics, 122–
      125
  ethical considerations, 128–129
Section 504 Accommodation Plan
  definition, 93
Self-care and self-determination in school
    nursing practice, 15

Skills, 93
Social and emotional school climate, 19
Social determinants of health
  definition, 93
Social services in school nursing practice,
    19
Special need students, 25–26
Staff wellness [2011], 125
Stakeholders
  definition, 93
Standards
  definition, 93
Standards of Practice, 17
Standards of Practice for School Nursing
    [2011]
  assessment, 7, 43–45, 120
    measurement criteria, 130
  consultation, 120
    measurement criteria, 141
  coordination of care, 8, 55–56, 120
    measurement criteria, 138
  diagnosis, 7, 46–47, 120
    measurement criteria, 132
  evaluation, 8, 59–60, 120
    measurement criteria, 143
  health teaching and health promotion,
      8, 57–58, 120
    measurement criteria, 139
  implementation, 8, 52–54, 120
    measurement criteria, 137
  outcomes identification, 8, 48–49, 120
    measurement criteria, 133
  planning, 8, 50–51, 120
    measurement criteria, 135
  prescriptive authority and treatment,
      120
    measurement criteria, 142
Standards of Professional Performance
    for School Nursing [2011]
  collaboration, 68–69, 121
    measurement criteria, 151
  collegiality, 121
    measurement criteria, 149
  communication, 9, 66–67
  culturally congruent practice, 8, 63–65
  education, 9, 72–73, 121
    measurement criteria, 147
  environmental health, 9, 82–83